Praise for **Up the Down Escalator**

"Lisa Doggett's thoughtful new mem— — — — and vital insights into a health care syste— — — — nind. As a family physician contending — — — — lt account of her struggles to sustain a — — — — own health challenges, and raises awareness for those who have been facing by the system's inequities. This book demands attention from those who seek a more just and compassionate world and want to understand how to make it so."

—**Stacey Abrams,** political leader, voting rights activist, and *New York Times* bestselling author

"Lisa Doggett writes candidly and with immense good humor and grace about her fears—for her health, her patients, her children, her husband—and her frustrations with same. She can be neurotic, unhappy, angry, but more than anything she is compassionate, strong, and always learning. To grab at our gut, a memoir must be fearless and unflinchingly honest. Funny helps, too. Doggett delivers, and how."

—**Julie Powell,** *New York Times* bestselling author of *Julie and Julia*

"A physician serving impoverished, uninsured patients, while coping with her own serious health problem, could be a story filled with darkness—but not this memoir. Instead, Dr. Lisa Doggett offers the consistent luminescence of compassion and hopefulness along with a much-needed vision for a more humane healthcare system. It is truly inspirational!"

—**Ron Pollack,** chair emeritus, formerly founding executive director, Families USA

"In vivid details, Dr. Doggett shares her experiences as clinician, mother, and wife through meaningful and intimate conversations, and personal monologues of internal thought processes and private emotional struggles. *Up the Down Escalator* is inspiring and uplifting, for those curious about physicians with their own health challenges or for those with the challenge of MS. But most all, Dr. Doggett's memoir speaks to all of us of that fragility of our human experience buoyed by the profound discovery of the power of our human spirit through love and our inner determination. A beautiful read!"

—**David W. Willis, MD, FAAP,** senior fellow, Center for the Study of Social Policy, director for the Nurture Connection Initiative

"To be heard, seen, and believed is what any person wants from a doctor. To have that doctor understand and share the exam table side of the doctor-patient relationship is rare and eye-opening. Lisa walks us through that progression in her career and personal life. A must read for doctors and patients alike."

—**Lisa Sailor,** MS and disability activist

Up the Down Escalator

MEDICINE, MOTHERHOOD, AND MULTIPLE SCLEROSIS

Lisa Doggett, MD

Health Communications, Inc.
Boca Raton, Florida

www.hcibooks.com

Author's note: While the events and stories depicted in this work are true, I have taken liberties with the timeline, dialogue, and details—gaps in my memory that can never be filled. To protect their privacy, I've disguised patients and created some patient composites. I've also changed the names and some identifying details of my doctors and certain others, as well as pharmacies and clinics.

Library of Congress Cataloging-in-Publication Data

Doggett, Lisa, author.
Up the down escalator: a doctor navigates disease and disorder / by
  Lisa Doggett, M.D.
Boca Raton, FL: Health Communications, Inc., [2023]
LCCN 2023006639 (print) | LCCN 2023006640 (ebook) |
ISBN 9780757324864 (paperback)
ISBN 075732486X (paperback)
ISBN 9780757324871 (epub)
ISBN 0757324878 (epub)
LCSH: Doggett, Lisa. | Doggett, Lisa—

Health. | Multiple sclerosis—Patients—Texas—Austin—Biography. Physicians—
  Texas—Austin—Biography. |

MEDICAL / Family & General Practice | BIOGRAPHY & AUTOBIOGRAPHY /
  Personal Memoirs

LCC RC377 .D635 2023 (print) | LCC RC377 (ebook) | DDC
  616.8/340092 [B]—dc23/eng/20230414

LC record available at https://lccn.loc.gov/2023006639
LC ebook record available at https://lccn.loc.gov/2023006640

Publisher: Health Communications, Inc.
        301 Crawford Boulevard, Suite 200
        Boca Raton, FL 33432-3762

Cover, interior design, and typesetting by Larissa Hise Henoch

From the Author

Thank you for reading my story. As I've discovered over nearly a decade and a half of living with multiple sclerosis and meeting many others with this strange disease, no two cases are the same. For those living with MS, some of my experiences may resonate with you. Others may not, and that's okay. This is not a how-to guide, but just one person's experience. I don't pretend to have all the answers. I still struggle with uncertainty, stress, and even rage, at times, over MS symptoms. And I don't know how to fix the U.S. health care system that continues to leave so many behind. I've grown a lot since my diagnosis, but I know I still have much to learn. My hope is that this narrative will provide validation for some of the challenges faced by those of you with chronic conditions and spark new insights to further your own growth. I hope it will help you power forward with courage and grace and let you know you are not alone.

For Don, Ella, and Clara,
whose laughter, love, and encouragement
have sustained me during dark days.
Thank you for joining me
on this journey.

Contents

CHAPTER 1

Mr. Sloane

February 1997

The man's arms and legs were shrunken, atrophied from disuse. His hands were twisted and stiff, curled into rigid fists. He moaned on the long, white stretcher. I stood in the corner, shifting my gaze to the window, the lights in the parking lot, and the dark sky beyond. He used to be a soldier.

"This is a fifty-six-year-old white male with a history of multiple sclerosis and hypertension," the second-year surgery resident said. "He developed acute, lower abdominal pain earlier today associated with vomiting. Exam reveals abdominal distension and diffuse tenderness to palpation."

"Okay, so what's your diagnosis?" Matt, the senior resident, asked.

"Well, obviously intestinal obstruction, uh, probably volvulus."

"Sounds like it," Matt exclaimed, his voice eager at the prospect of operating.

Volvulus—an abnormal twisting of the intestine back on itself—can cause a logjam in the abdomen. The obstruction blocks the passage of waste products and can cause severe tissue damage, infection, and death. It's a bread-and-butter diagnosis in general surgery, but in the weeks since starting my required surgery rotation at the Veterans Affairs Hospital in Houston, I'd only read about it in my medical school textbook.

"Oh, God, please help!" our patient cried out.

"Yeah, hey, can we get him some more morphine?" Matt ordered a nurse nearby. Then he turned to me. "Did you examine this guy?"

I recoiled at the thought. An exam would hurt, and this "learning opportunity" for me didn't seem worth the price of further pain. But I knew better than to question the rigid chain of command that framed my medical education.

"Hi, Mr. Sloane," I whispered, gently touching the man's shoulder. "I'm Lisa, one of the medical students. I'm so sorry you're hurting. We just need to check your belly once more."

He moaned again, but he rolled onto his back to allow me to examine him.

"The nurse is getting more pain meds right now," I said, helping to readjust his sheet and blanket, trying to keep most of him covered as I exposed the parts I needed to assess.

"Come on," the second-year resident interrupted. "We've gotta get this guy to radiology."

"Sorry, Mr. Sloane." I placed my stethoscope over the patient's abdomen, listening for the familiar little squeaks and gurgles that indicate a healthy and active intestinal system. Nothing. I pushed down slightly, pulling back my hand as his abdomen tightened. He winced.

"Absent bowel sounds," I said to the resident. "And he has guarding."

Even I could tell Mr. Sloane had an obstruction.

But the resident wasn't listening.

"Come on . . . hustle, hustle," he said, waving his arms as if to push me aside. He grabbed the metal sidebar of the stretcher and pushed it up into place.

I jumped out of the way, thankful to see the nurse injecting more morphine into Mr. Sloane's IV. Within seconds, he relaxed a little.

Sneaking a glance at my watch, I calculated the hours I had been at the hospital: almost eighteen. Every one of my bones, muscles, and ligaments was tired. Calcaneus, talus, navicular, cuboid . . . I had learned all the bones in the foot, and each of them screamed for a break. My day had started at 6:00 AM with hospital rounds. After visiting the four patients assigned to me and writing short notes, I had trotted behind the surgery residents as we stopped by to check on patients under the care of our team: Mr. Rossi had been delirious overnight and pulled out his IV. Mr. Peterson was asking for more pain medicines. Mr. Visiago's wound was healing well, and he might go home.

A morning conference about the management of pancreatitis allowed me to sit for thirty minutes, but I spent hours standing after that, watching two hernia repairs, a splenectomy, and a longer vascular bypass procedure to improve blood flow to an ischemic (oxygen-deprived) foot. Lunch was pizza in the break room, gulped down between surgeries. Dinner—at 9:00 PM—was cold pizza left over from lunch. The day was endless, and I was tired. Tired of standing in place, watching as bodies were cut open and blood suctioned. Tired of the stale air polluted by the smell of burning flesh from the cautery pen. Tired of beeping IV poles and dirty jokes.

I was also ashamed. Mr. Sloane was suffering. He was in the hospital, without any family, being poked and prodded a few extra times for the benefit of my education. He felt like his insides were exploding, yet I was bemoaning my sore legs and inevitable sleep deprivation. *How self-absorbed of me.*

I was also trying to impress the more senior members of my team. I was programmed to seek their approval. I had always been driven to work hard and study hard, but medical school had humbled me. It wasn't so easy to excel here. Even if I could cope with the long hours and respect the strict hierarchy, there was just so much to learn.

During operations, the residents would grill me on my knowledge of anatomy—never my strong suit—and laugh in my surgically masked face if I didn't answer correctly.

"What's this artery?" the resident would ask, lifting a thin pink cord with the tiny laparoscopic tool during a gallbladder surgery, his harsh voice muffled.

"The hepatic artery?" I'd guess.

"God, no! It's the anterior branch of the cystic artery. Remember Calot's triangle? How many times have we gone over this?"

I wasn't used to being incompetent. But no matter how many times I reviewed the illustrations in my textbook, I had trouble identifying the arteries, veins, and other anatomic structures during an operation. There was no glue in my brain for the intricate details of human anatomy.

I trailed behind as a hospital orderly wheeled the stretcher to the radiology department. When the elevator door opened to the basement hallway, the second-year resident bounded out, followed by the attendant with the stretcher and finally me, marveling at the resident's enthusiasm and trying to ignore every impulse to slouch to the floor.

At the end of a short corridor, we turned into a room about the same size as a standard patient room, except with a large x-ray machine instead of a hospital bed. The machine loomed over a metal table covered with a white pad and sheet and illuminated by the glare of fluorescent lights. It was nearly midnight.

White and gray, I thought. Except for the sea-foam scrubs and the blue surgical gowns we wore, the hospital was devoid of color, almost like an old movie. Blood was the other exception.

"So, is there a connection between this guy's MS and volvulus?" the second-year resident asked me while the techs started preparing Mr. Sloane for a barium enema.

"Yes?" I answered, hoping I was right.

"Correct. MS increases his risk. And what are the other risk factors?"

I didn't know. "Uh, older age?" Older age is a risk factor for nearly everything; it was a calculated guess.

The resident nodded. "Older age, chronic constipation, laxative abuse, other neurologic and psychiatric conditions," he recited. He must have memorized the textbook.

"So, we're gonna do the enema procedure first to confirm the diagnosis," he said. "Sometimes that'll straighten out the twisted intestine, but the patient will almost certainly need surgery after that to keep it from happening again. He may bleed. Then we'll definitely have to operate."

Mr. Sloane shouted out once more in pain, as the orderlies moved him onto the thin pad on top of the metal table. He was tangled in the bed linens, and I could see his boney spine through the sheet. His suffering was acute and heavy. Intrigued and repelled, I wanted to comfort him, and I wanted to run from the room. But I was an obedient student, and I waited. The enema would confirm volvulus. If the patient agreed, we would operate. If all went as planned, we would return him to his usual state of health or, in his case, to his usual state of severe, chronic, painful suffering. Even if we fixed the obstruction, there was no cure for his MS.

I stood nearby, watching as this broken man was helped into a fetal-like position while a tube was inserted into his rectum. I imagined that once, decades before, he was young and vibrant. Maybe he liked the Doors and played basketball. Maybe he built houses or worked in a restaurant. Then he went to Vietnam. Did he leave behind a girlfriend, or a young wife and child who celebrated his return? I thought of him coming home, with big hopes for his future, only to have his plans sabotaged by MS, to have his body forsake him.

My life had been sheltered before this surgery rotation. I had been spared such sights, such intimate connection with misery. Growing up in Austin, I lived with my parents and sister in a two-story house with a front yard big enough for Slip 'N Slides and games of freeze tag. My grandparents lived two miles away, and we visited every weekend. Everyone was healthy; we liked each other and got along. No car accidents, violent fights, surprise cancer diagnoses.

I felt an urge to talk to Don, my boyfriend since college and a fellow medical student. I wanted to tell him about Mr. Sloane's case, to process this random cruelty. I wanted his help to understand this terrible disease that destroyed a man's life and left him with a potentially fatal surgical condition. I wanted his reassurance: Mr. Sloane's condition was rare. Maybe he would be okay. Don also might remind me that we had chosen to be doctors to help people, and we were learning how to do just that.

But it was too late to call. Don would be asleep.

When Mr. Sloane's procedure was over, I returned to the break room, picked up my textbook, and settled down on an ancient couch to read about volvulus.

I don't remember if I bid good night to Mr. Sloane, but I can imagine slipping by his room a little later, after I finally was sent to the call room for a couple hours of precious sleep before morning rounds. He was the first patient I had seen not only with volvulus but MS: the instigator of his abdominal obstruction and the cause of his devastating decline. I would have been relieved to see him sleeping, despite the glare of the vital signs monitor. "I hope you don't bleed. I hope you don't need surgery," I might have whispered. "You've been through enough."

CHAPTER 2

Caring for Our Own

October 2009

I looked down at the intake form and the reason for this new patient's visit to the clinic near downtown Austin where I served as director: electrocution.

Mauricio was a recent Mexican immigrant in his early fifties. He had sustained severe electrical burns over 40 percent of his body while repairing high-voltage power lines. After a two-month hospitalization, he was now home but uninsured and unable to work, walk, or even speak normally. As I collected a basic medical history, I noticed the worn cuffs of his shirt sleeves, the stains on his wife's faded pink dress. This family was struggling.

"*Doctora*, he's in pain all the time," Mauricio's wife said in Spanish, holding back tears.

Mauricio mumbled something that I couldn't understand.

"What's that?" I asked, leaning closer to his wheelchair.

"*Me duele, y no puedo dormir*," he said more clearly. (I hurt, and I can't sleep.)

I could only imagine. His right forearm and the side of his neck were scarred, discolored from the burns. I didn't know how I could possibly help.

"It's good you're here," I said in passable but imperfect Spanish. I wanted him to feel welcome, even if there wasn't much I could do. "What's bothering you the most today?"

"My legs and back," Mauricio answered. His dark hair was streaked with gray. He sat almost motionless, staring at the floor.

"And he has diabetes," his wife added. "His sugars are always high."

I met her timid gaze, noting her sad brown eyes, her dark hair pulled back in a low bun at the nape of her neck. I nodded. "Okay, well, I think I can help you with that." If nothing else, at least I knew how to take care of diabetes.

Mauricio had been discharged from the hospital three weeks before with almost no plan for follow-up care. He and his wife had been all over the city trying to find a doctor who could see him without insurance. He'd been in and out of the emergency room and was receiving bills for tens of thousands of dollars, which he could never pay. Finally, they had landed at our small family medicine clinic. We charged patients on a sliding scale, but most of our funding came from a local university, grants from the state, local foundations, and a partnership with the city's community clinic system. We were there to care for patients like Mauricio, who had run out of other options.

"Do you have family that can help you?" I asked.

"Our son lives in California. The rest are in Mexico," his wife said.

"What about friends, a church?" I asked.

"No," she said, looking away.

"What about the burn clinic? Can you go back there?" I asked.

"*Sí*," Mauricio's wife said, "we have an appointment there next week."

Thank God.

"But they only give medicines for his pain and check his burns," she added. "They don't help with anything else."

My physical exam was limited by Mauricio's mobility constraints, but I got a sense of the damage. Both legs and one arm had been badly burned. He had received multiple skin grafts that appeared to be healing well, but the nerve damage that left him partially paralyzed was probably irreversible.

"Have you applied for disability?" I asked.

"We don't have documents." Mauricio's wife looked away, embarrassed. She meant that they were in the country illegally, a situation I was used to, and one that limited our options further.

"What about workers' comp?" I asked.

"No, he didn't work for a company," Mauricio's wife said.

I gathered that he was some sort of contractor, though I never figured out how or why he was working on high-voltage power lines. A lot of my patients were like Mauricio. They cobbled together a living from odd jobs in construction or landscaping or whatever else came their way via the unofficial day-labor spot in front of the Home Depot. It was a hard way to pay the bills, and it left them vulnerable to all manner of accidents, cruel employers who withheld wages, and landlords who refused to fix broken pipes or get rid of rats. Most were Hispanic, like Mauricio—doubly challenged by language barriers and almost certainly racism, sometimes oblique, sometimes more overt.

"Let's start by getting some lab work," I said. "We can do that today. I also want to get the records from the hospital and the burn clinic.

We can also check into options for physical therapy . . . but it may be expensive."

I turned to walk out of the room but stopped, struck again by the immense sadness and hopelessness of the situation. A tiny blunder, a miscalculation, and a life was ruined. I turned and went back to Mauricio, squatting down next to him, placing my hand on the cold sidebar of the wheelchair. I felt a little awkward and uncomfortable, but I couldn't walk out without saying something more, wholly inadequate as it would be. "I am so sorry this happened to you." I stood up again, putting a hand on his wife's arm. "I'm sorry."

After seven years of work as a family physician for people without private insurance, I was accustomed to tragedy. The protective bubble of my childhood had been popped long before, during my grueling medical training. Bat-infested apartments, deported spouses, runaway children, and freak accidents were all part of a day's work. Mental illness and chronic disease were endemic.

Health insurance was unattainable for many of my patients. Eligibility for Medicaid, a joint federal and state program that provides health coverage to some people with low incomes, was more restricted in Texas than in many other states. Nonpregnant adults didn't (and still don't) qualify, unless they were disabled or had children and very low incomes. The Affordable Care Act, passed in 2010, with most major provisions phased in by 2014, extended coverage to millions of people, dropping the uninsured rate in the United States among non-elderly individuals from 17.8 percent in 2010 to 10.2 percent in 2021.[1] But even had it existed earlier, it wouldn't have helped many of my patients, given Texas's failure to expand Medicaid coverage to adults who earn up to 138 percent of the federal poverty level. To those like

Mauricio, who were undocumented, health insurance was completely out of reach.

Being uninsured was—and still is—a risk factor for poor health outcomes. Compared to those with health coverage, people without insurance have more fragmented medical care and lower rates of preventive screening tests. They are significantly more likely to die early. A 2012 report by Families USA stated that between 2005 and 2010, the number of premature deaths each year due to a lack of health coverage rose from 20,350 to 26,100.[2] Such disparities were compounded years later by the global pandemic. A 2022 study estimated that, had it existed, universal health care from the beginning of the pandemic until mid-March 2022 could have prevented over 338,000 deaths from COVID.[3]

Some of our patients qualified for the city's Medical Access Program—a sort of health insurance alternative for those below a certain income threshold. But many had to pay for much or all of their health care costs. While our clinic didn't turn anyone away based on ability to pay, our patients struggled to afford their medications and access specialty care. In other words, they could see me for free, if necessary, but if they needed anything else—radiology services, medicines, referrals to other doctors—they often had to foot the bill.

In the years since I had begun working in community clinics, I'd learned to navigate the highways, side streets, and dark, crooked alleyways of Austin's health care system. There were sharp turns and frequent dead ends. Still, I knew the discount pharmacies and the ones that overcharged. I could rattle off long lists of generic medicines that I favored over the expensive new drugs preferred by physicians in private practice. I also had a mental Rolodex of specialty doctors I could call for favors: the dermatologist who would review pictures of rashes by e-mail, the gastroenterologist who would give me advice over the phone for patients with cirrhosis of the liver, the hand surgeon who would see my patients for free.

Despite my familiarity with the underground network of supports for people without insurance, I had been an unlikely candidate for the job of clinic director. Two years before, when I interviewed for the position, I was pregnant with my second child, and I already had a toddler at home who served as a fine distraction from work, from everything. I had practiced for five years at a similar clinic for uninsured patients, but I had no management experience, no clue how to hire staff, review budgets, or do performance evaluations. As for running a medical practice, especially a new clinic with no infrastructure and unreliable funding—let's just say it was a reach. But when several other more suitable applicants turned down the director position, I got the job by default, in spite of my deficiencies. I was thrilled—and scared that I couldn't live up to the task. My family congratulated me. My dad, a U.S. Congressman, was proud. I was adding to our legacy of public service. Only looking back did I realize there may have been a reason—many reasons—why no one else wanted that job.

Be careful what you wish for.

The learning curve at the clinic had been more than steep; it was practically vertical. I marveled that I still had the job two years later. I was now supported by a competent team of committed, mission-driven women. My nurse and office manager, Kim, had a bad-ass toughness and eye for detail. Half Korean and half white, she had learned Spanish and spent much of her day on the phone, communicating in whichever language was needed, with patients in crisis or chasing down medical records from various hospitals. Sara Maria, originally from South Texas, was a skilled bilingual medical assistant who sometimes guessed a patient's diagnosis before I did. Terri, a wondrous nurse practitioner, shared an office with me. Well loved by patients and colleagues, Terri—a slim, white woman twenty years my senior—worked harder than anyone. She also laughed at my jokes and could coax me out of grumpy moods that I sometimes brought to work. Other staff included a part-time endocrinologist, women's health nurse practitioner, receptionist, and other medical assistants. Two years after assuming the monumental task of directing the clinic, I alternated between pride in what I'd built and terror that at any second it could collapse.

Like Mauricio, my next patient, Faith, was ready to challenge my resourcefulness and creative problem-solving skills.

"I'm so sorry, Dr. Doggett, but I couldn't get the chest x-ray," she said before I could greet her.

"Oh? What happened?" I asked, settling on my stool near her chair. I knew Faith well by now. Due to the severity of her asthma, we had seen each other often over the last several months.

"The hospital says I owe them six hundred dollars from the last set of x-rays I had for my knees," she explained. "I can't get the chest x-ray until I pay for the knee x-rays."

"Six hundred dollars? That's ridiculous. I would think they should have cost about sixty or seventy dollars—definitely less than a hundred."

"No. I've got the letter right here."

She handed me a crumbled piece of paper, confirming the price: $623.

I sighed and looked at her. "This is totally unreasonable, ridiculous."

Faith's lack of insurance was the problem. The hospital was inflating her bill, with no regard to her financial situation. As an individual, she didn't have the clout to negotiate lower rates like an insurance company, which could arrange for steep discounts.

Faith wasn't alone—nor has the situation improved. A *Wall Street Journal* analysis published in 2021 showed that hospitals often charge uninsured patients the highest prices. Across 1,166 hospitals included in the report, for example, the fees for uninsured patients were 3.6 times higher than the average rates paid by health plans covering people enrolled in Medicare Advantage.[4] Faith had gone to the public hospital, presumably her best and cheapest option, but they were still ripping her off.

"What should I do? I can't pay this bill," she said.

"Let me make a copy of that, and we'll give them a call," I said. "How are you doing other than that?"

To my relief, Faith told me her asthma was better. Kim had helped find a discount pharmacy where she had refilled her inhalers. Her knee pain had improved as well.

I adored this patient and felt tremendous sympathy for her. In addition to early-onset arthritis and thyroid problems, Faith had the worst asthma I'd ever seen. Because her asthma limited her activities and required oral as well as inhaled steroids, she continued to gain weight, restricting her further. She was forty years old and a nonsmoker, yet every breath was an effort. Even on her good days, Faith wheezed and struggled. Getting out of a chair, lying down, getting dressed— everything was exhausting and exceedingly difficult. She needed to be examined by a specialist at the public hospital's asthma clinic, but they wouldn't see her until she had another chest x-ray. Even with the chest x-ray, she'd have to wait months for her appointment.

I listened to her lungs, which sounded better than usual, though still noisy with scattered wheezes. We talked again about weight-loss strategies, and I refilled two of her medicines. I made myself a note to call the hospital and follow up with her later. I would have to pour precious minutes, maybe hours, into her case to confirm my suspicions about the expensive x-rays, and I would need more time to search for resources for Mauricio.

I resented the fact that I wouldn't get credit for any of this time from our funders or clinic administrators, who tallied and averaged the numbers of patient visits each day to assess my "productivity," pressuring me to fit in more and more visits. And I resented our fee-for-service health care system that valued quantity over quality, and procedures—biopsies, surgeries, colonoscopies—over face-to-face time and the thinking part of medicine.

Most of all, I was enraged by the endless barriers that kept Faith, Mauricio, and so many others from ever getting healthy. My home state of Texas ranked dead last in the United States for the number of residents covered by health insurance. We had impressive highways, NASA, the biggest rodeo, and the tallest capitol building. We had no state income tax. In Houston, we had the largest medical center in the world, where I went to medical school. Yet we failed to care for our own.

I couldn't dwell on these injustices or on Faith. I had to move on. As usual, I was falling behind.

My next two patients were pleasant women, both in their fifties, chatty and friendly, both with diabetes and high blood pressure. I made minor adjustments in their medication regimens, discussing back pain with one and vague muscle aches with the other.

My fifth patient was a no-show. Our patient population was notorious for failing to keep appointments. The reasons ranged from lack of childcare or transportation to family obligations to an unaccommodating boss to sometimes just plain forgetting. It was unfortunate, but they were pulled in so many directions. Personal health care just wasn't the top priority.

Still, that uncertainty added to everyone's stress at the clinic. We would schedule a manageable number of patients for the morning, and then only three would show up. So we would add more slots, and the next day everyone would show up, and the first three patients would be depressed men with testicular pain and six other problems each. That afternoon I was thankful for the no-show because I was almost an hour behind and needed to catch up. But it meant one less visit on our monthly tally. We were continuing to fall short of productivity expectations, since we were unable to see as many patients as our funders and partners expected. The number of patient visits was the most important measure of our worth—more important than what was accomplished during those visits, patient satisfaction, health outcomes, or anything else. Our failure jeopardized our funding and the clinic's very existence.

Always on the lookout for ways to care for our patients while keeping an eye on our productivity goals, Kim, Sara Maria, and I tried to restrict each patient to just one or two problems. "What is the main reason you're here today?" Sara Maria would ask when bringing someone back to the exam room. If the patient listed multiple complaints, Sara Maria would offer to schedule a future appointment to address issues of lower priority. But despite her attempt to focus my next visit on one or two concerns, the patient, Connie, had insisted we discuss her breathing difficulties, leg pain, headaches, insomnia, and nausea.

I had seen Connie three or four times before. A white woman in her early sixties, she had never finished high school, dropping out, perhaps, to care for a sick family member or help cover the rent by getting a job. Twice divorced, she now lived alone. She was crying when I entered the room.

"Hey," I said, suppressing a cough. The room smelled of smoke. She hadn't been able to quit. "What's going on?"

"I can't . . . my son . . . my son is in prison," she managed, brushing away dark hair, revealing smeared mascara around her eyes. Blue eyes. Her eyes were blue like mine.

"Oh, Connie . . ." My mind bolted, imagining a child in prison. Frustration and disappointment, the constant fear for his safety, a stark cell with no privacy, no beauty. I needed to stay on task and keep Connie focused. One of us had to keep it together. I decided not to ask for any details but to try to steer her back to the medical appointment.

"I'm so sorry. It makes it hard to take care of yourself when you're dealing with a stressful situation like that," I said. It felt like such a pat thing to say, but I had to move on to the real reasons for her visit. "How are things going with your breathing?"

I had concluded after her first visit that the "asthma" she described was more likely chronic obstructive pulmonary disease (COPD), which resulted from her smoking. The diseases are similar, but treatments differ. Either way she needed to lay off the cigarettes. Easier said than done.

"I'm not doing so good."

"Did you start the new inhaler we talked about last time?"

"Yes, but it made my leg hurt, so I stopped. I'm using that other one now," she said, having calmed down a bit. She pulled out a tissue from a denim handbag and wiped the mascara from under her eyes.

"The albuterol?" I asked, referring to the inhaler we use on an as-needed basis for people with asthma and COPD.

"I think so."

"How often are you needing it?" I asked. I was trying to determine if she really needed the other inhaler, a daily "controller," to reduce her symptoms.

"I don't know. It depends. I use it when I get the breathing trouble."

"How often is that?"

"If I get the coughing, I use it sometimes," she said. She pulled at a loose thread on her bag. I could see the pack of Marlboros just inside the top.

"Are you needing the albuterol more than twice a week?" It was a simple question, and her answer, if I could get one, would help determine if she needed another medicine.

"Oh, I use it a lot."

"More than twice a week?" I didn't know how long I could mask my impatience.

"I think maybe a couple times a day," she finally conceded.

"Okay, that's a lot. Too much."

Indeed, the other inhaler, the controller, was necessary.

"I don't think the other inhaler is causing your leg pain," I said. "I think that's a different issue we need to discuss. Actually, are you still having the leg pain?"

"Yes, especially when I have to walk a lot. My car broke so I'm having to take the bus."

"Well, if you stopped the inhaler, and you're still having the leg pain, the inhaler probably isn't causing the leg pain." I paused, hoping that remark would sink in. "I think we should either try that inhaler again, or I can write you a prescription for something else."

She agreed to restart the same inhaler. We then went on to discuss her headaches and insomnia (stress-related, most likely), nausea (which sounded more like acid reflux), and the leg pain, which correlated with the broken car and increased walking. I gave her a flier for a low-cost counseling center where she could talk to someone more about her son, the car situation, and her various stresses. They could assess her more thoroughly for depression, which I strongly suspected. I hoped she would call for an appointment. Only afterward did I realize that I had failed to address the root cause of her breathing issues: smoking. It was an unfortunate oversight but would have to wait until her next visit in a few weeks.

I struggled through one more appointment, explaining to my last patient that the "spider bite" he revealed on his lower abdomen actually was an abscess, then I pulled in Sara Maria to assist as I drained it. That appointment took longer than the allotted time as well, but at least no one else was waiting.

At last, I was done. It always felt like an enormous achievement to finish another day at the clinic. Unpredictable and rushed, punctuated by moments of unbearable sadness and rare celebrations of success, my work was a paradox, leaving me fulfilled and drained at the same time. With amusement, I recalled a conversation back in medical school when I talked to another student about choosing family medicine as my specialty. "Family medicine is kind of boring," she said. "It's a bunch of coughs and colds."

If only.

In reality, I would have been bored in a clinic without challenges. I enjoyed the aha moments of discovery: diagnosing an overactive thyroid in a patient with anxiety and weight loss, finding vitamin B12 deficiency in someone with anemia and fatigue. Forever frustrated with the limits facing my patients, I still relished the victories when I succeeded in helping someone get free cholesterol medicine through a pharmaceutical company's patient assistance program, access low-cost dental care, or get caught up on long-overdue immunizations.

Care for underserved populations was not formally recognized as its own medical specialty. To practice in a community clinic, I didn't have to take a test beyond my board exams to be a family physician. Nor did I have to complete a fellowship in community health. Providing care for people without insurance, though, required a resourcefulness and mindset that went beyond what was needed in some more traditional settings. In practice, it was its own specialty, like cardiology or oncology.

If only the successes weren't far outnumbered by the defeats. If only the time pressure, the stress of always running late, the paperwork, and the communication barriers didn't leave me perpetually overwhelmed. So much of my job satisfaction, if I could even call it that, was that sense of relief after completing another clinic session.

But as I settled down at my desk to finish writing my patient care notes, I reflected on the afternoon of bouncing from crisis to crisis. It was a privilege to jump into the fire with my patients, to face the suffocating problems that brought them into my office. Just to be there, together, as you're going through hell. I only had to sit with them for a short time, and it was hard to do, but it was important—often more important than the x-rays, the medicines, and the lab tests. I was fortunate that I could jump out again and return to a life where the biggest problems were two fussy kids, a too-busy pediatrician husband, and too little sleep.

CHAPTER 3

The Tall Guy at MIT

November 1991

A fraternity party at MIT? It seemed like an oxymoron. A prestigious academic mecca, the Massachusetts Institute of Technology was a school for brilliant young people seeking PhDs and Nobel Prizes. The students, I assumed, spent their time doing physics experiments, solving impossible math problems, and watching *Star Trek*. It wasn't the sort of place that had fraternities. Or frat parties.

I had reunited with two high school friends, Melissa and Dalit, for the weekend. All of us, recent graduates of McCallum High School in Austin and now freshmen at East Coast colleges, were gathered for a girls' weekend in Boston. Dalit knew a guy at MIT.

I didn't want to go to the party. It had been a perfect autumn day, wandering through Boston and Cambridge. Dressed in oversized sweaters and jackets, Melissa, Dalit, and I posed for pictures in

23

Quincy Market, smiling and squinting in the sunshine, overjoyed to be back together, now as college women. We relished our freedom to explore this new city, without having to check in with parents or anyone. I was learning to row and bought a crew poster at the Harvard bookstore and a Head of the Charles rowing shirt. We had dinner at Legal Seafood. Now I was ready to head back to Melissa's dorm, make popcorn, and watch a movie. *Madonna: Truth or Dare* had just come out on video, and I was dying to see it. I had no interest in a fraternity party, but I didn't have an acceptable alternate plan, and I wanted to be with my friends, so the party it was.

A tall guy, holding a plate of pasta in one hand, opened the door and welcomed us into the historic brownstone on Beacon Street. I didn't catch his name. He turned to call Dalit's friend, yelling up the stairwell, "Mark! Front door!"

We followed him into the house and waited in the entryway as he presumably went to look for Mark. Although I was grateful to be out of the cold, I was uncomfortable. I had never set foot in a fraternity house. It wasn't my scene, and I wanted to leave. More guys were hanging out in the nearby living room, eating dinner, and watching *Star Trek: The Next Generation.* At least I got that part right.

The party hadn't started yet—they hadn't even brought in a keg, not that I wanted any beer. I didn't want to watch *Star Trek* either, though Dalit and Melissa joined Mark, once he had been located, near the TV. Instead, I asked for a quiet place to work. One of the guys showed me the Chapter Room.

"This is where we have meetings, but no one will bother you if you wanna hang out here," he said.

I settled on the leather couch to read a book for my Native American Studies class. The room was old-school Boston meets frat house:

wood paneling and bay windows, overstuffed chairs and dried vomit on the floor. I was glad to sit alone and dive back into the life of Mary Brave Bird on the South Dakota reservation. I settled in for a while, but at some point, *Star Trek* must have ended, and my friends found me for a tour of the house.

Melissa caught sight of my book, and as I stuffed it back into my shopping bag, I whispered, "I know. . . . You don't have to say it. I'm the biggest nerd here."

Dalit's friend, Mark, guided us through the living quarters, room by room. We wandered through, mesmerized. The house was the dream of adolescent boys building their forts in the forest, but with real timber and sound construction, in the middle of the Back Bay. Each room was an impressive collage of creative engineering, no two remotely the same.

"Oh my God. This place is crazy!" I said, ducking under a platform to see the workspace below two beds near the ceiling. Violating every conceivable fire code, the guys had constructed lofts and caves in each room, taking advantage of the high ceilings and refining their work every summer.

We continued our tour, ending up in a triple bedroom at the end of a long hallway. The room, called "Deli Cheese," was bright with overhead lights and a couple of lamps. It had bunk beds at one end of the long, thin room, and at the other end was a loft with a waterbed. Through a large window, we could see lights reflected off the Charles River and the MIT campus beyond. The space below the beds was furnished with a sofa and desks. I saw the guy who had first greeted us and introduced myself.

"Oh yeah, I let you in earlier. I'm Donny. Or Don—either way," he said.

We had to look up at him—way up. My head barely came to his shoulder.

"How tall are you?" Dalit asked.

"Six-foot-seven," he said. He'd heard this question a few times before.

"Wow. Do you play basketball?" I asked.

"I did in high school. Not here, though. It takes a lot of time I didn't think I'd have."

What a nice guy. His tone was friendly and warm. I'm sure these conversations about his height and basketball got old, but he played along well and still seemed interested in talking to us. He wasn't flirting, though. He was genuine, even a little shy, and didn't seem to have an ulterior motive.

I wondered how I had been so oblivious that I didn't notice when he greeted us at the door. He had a kind, handsome face and dark brown hair. Usually, I would have been intimidated talking to a guy who was so attractive, but I felt comfortable with him.

While Dalit and Melissa talked to Mark, Donny and I exchanged the required demographic information. Me: Austin, Texas; freshman; Amherst College; unknown major—maybe political science and premed? Him: Scranton, Pennsylvania; sophomore; MIT; chemistry major, maybe premed.

Then a ninety-degree turn: "Was I seeing things, or did I almost step on a lizard before?" I asked. It had struck me as odd to see a tiny reptile on the fourth floor of this Boston residence, but then again, nothing about the place was normal.

"Yeah, we had a roach problem, so we got gecko lizards," Donny said.

Geckos to solve the roach problem? It took me a second to figure it out. "Oh, you mean you got lizards to eat them? Seriously?"

"It was either that or call an exterminator," Donny smiled. "It actually seems to have worked. Not many roaches."

Introductions and lizard stories out of the way, Mark suggested a game of Twister. I couldn't remember the last time I had played, but I was in. Donny begged off and sat against the wall leafing through the latest edition of *Rolling Stone*.

Right hand, red. Left foot, yellow. I laughed with the others as we took turns contorting ourselves like Cirque du Soleil wannabes and then falling down when the combination of colors, hands, and feet became impossible. But I kept glancing at Donny. He seemed absorbed in the magazine, but I thought I caught him looking in my direction once or twice.

When the silly, short-lived game ended, I got up the nerve to join him.

"What's the best album of the year?" Donny asked as I approached.

"I don't know. Why?"

"There's this survey. A reader's poll," he said, holding up the magazine.

"Oh, a poll—like for best band? Maybe I could help," I said, sitting down next to him on an old couch under one of the loft beds. I felt self-conscious, half wanting to retreat back into the Chapter Room with my book. He was out of my league. But I would probably never see him again, so what the hell?

"What kinds of music do you like anyway?" I asked.

"Mostly classic rock," he said, "but lots of new stuff right now is good, too—Nirvana, Pearl Jam. That new REM album—have you heard of it? *Out of Time*? It's really good."

Okay, so Donny didn't need any help from me.

"Nirvana, yeah," I said. "I feel like someone's always playing that song in my dorm, 'Smells Like Teen Spirit.'"

I was glad I knew the names of the bands he was talking about. Even though I didn't read *Rolling Stone*, music was a pretty safe topic for me, far better than professional sports or TV shows.

"You probably know U2 has a new album coming out," Donny said. "It's being released tomorrow at midnight. Tower Records is just down the street. A few of us are going to get it as soon as it goes on sale."

His enthusiasm was contagious. Suddenly, I wanted to go with him to Tower Records to buy the album at midnight. Too bad Amherst College was two hours away.

Not only did he listen to music, I learned, but he played it, too. He had both an acoustic and electric guitar. He knew songs by Led Zeppelin, Pink Floyd, James Taylor. And although his passion was for rock music, he was genuinely impressed when I told him that I played the piano: Chopin, Debussy, Mozart.

"You've played for thirteen years?" he said. "I bet you're really good. I'd love to hear you sometime."

I didn't see how that would ever be possible, but I smiled at the thought.

Melissa and Dalit interrupted us. They were ready to leave, just as most people were arriving.

"We've got to catch the bus back to my dorm," Melissa said.

We weren't partiers anyway, and I didn't protest. But before I left, Donny surprised me with an unusual request.

"We should exchange e-mail addresses," he said.

"What? E-mail?" *Did I even know my e-mail address?*

"Yeah, do you have e-mail? It's pretty cool. I write my high school friend at Penn every few days," he said.

"I haven't really used it much, but yeah, I have it," I said.

I jotted my e-mail address on a piece of scratch paper, and Donny did the same.

I never expected to hear from him again. I remember remarking to Dalit and Melissa, "That guy, Donny, was pretty cute," but I thought that was the end of it. Our encounter had been brief, and we didn't even go to school in the same city.

When I saw an e-mail from him a few days later, I felt surprised—and a spark of hope. I laughed at his description of the chaotic party that ensued after we left the fraternity house. He said he hoped I would return.

One e-mail turned into dozens as we cheered each other on through fall semester exams. We wrote letters over the winter break since we didn't have e-mail at home. Then we talked on the phone, deciding we should, in fact, see each other again. In January, Donny took the Peter Pan bus line to Amherst for a weekend. And that was it.

Ten years later, after supporting each other through medical school and residency, we were married.

A few years after that, we were a family of four.

CHAPTER 4

Worthy Pursuits

October 2009

The lake beckoned. I couldn't stay away, and I didn't want to run anywhere else. Austin's Lady Bird Lake, named after former first lady Lady Bird Johnson, stretches through downtown. It's a beloved feature of the city, with well-used trails and parks along its banks. Before having my two daughters, I had the time and freedom to hit the trail almost every morning. I'd drive from my house—just a few minutes away—and jog around the three-mile loop, sometimes with my mom or dad, always with my lanky lab mix, Mocha. Now I mostly ran on weekends, usually pushing a hardy jogging stroller from REI loaded with a kid or two.

On a Sunday in mid-October, I was excited to find a rare opportunity to run, child-free, with my new friend, Jess. She met me by the footbridge, across the street from Austin High School.

"I can't believe we managed this," I said as we took off, with Mocha leading the way.

"I know. I barely even know what to do with my arms when I'm not carrying a kid," she said, laughing.

We had met the year before when Jess's son, who was just two days older than my firstborn, Ella, joined our preschool class. We discovered our younger daughters were close in age as well, and soon we were meeting for playdates at the park and chatting at birthday parties. While our kids entertained one another, we bonded over shared political views and a love of books and travel. Jess stayed home with her children, and I envied her extra family time—the creative craft projects she organized, her midweek hikes with the kids. She offered a glimpse at another life path, one that was a little less hectic but still included the same child-rearing challenges—bedtime routines, picky eaters, temper tantrums. I appreciated her perspective and respected her different choice. I was grateful to our kids for inadvertently bringing us together.

We crossed the lake and jogged along its south side where the trail cut through the green, expansive Zilker Park, delighting in the cooler weather and sharing Halloween plans: a pumpkin-carving party, a school carnival. As we crossed another footbridge and ran by Zach Scott Theater, a woman raced past with an Austin Marathon T-shirt.

"I guess people are starting to train for the marathon now," I said. "It's like in February or something, right?"

"I think so," Jess said.

"That's twenty-six miles, I think. Can you even imagine?" I asked. "I could never do that."

We proceeded to list all the marathon runners we knew: a fellow mom from our preschool class, two friends from medical school, a former babysitter. I was in awe of them all. But I couldn't join them. I knew my limits.

"I'll have to satisfy myself with directing the clinic, raising my kids, and running the three-mile loop," I said.

"All worthy pursuits," my friend assured me.

c⁓

I doubted one of those pursuits—my career choice—the next day when I saw my schedule. "Oh God, I have to see *both* Belinda and Ms. Morris today?" I complained to Sara Maria.

Despite our new electronic medical record (EMR) system, large clumps of papers—radiology reports, prescription refill requests, old medical records—were stacked on my desk on either side, almost blocking the picture of Don, Ella, and our younger daughter, Clara. It would be a while before I could review and sign them so that they could be scanned into the electronic chart, though. First, I had patients to see.

"Belinda is already waiting," said Sara Maria. "She smells like smoke."

"What? She swore she'd never smoke again." I sighed. I knew how hard it was to give up smoking, but she had been doing so well.

"She's embarrassed to tell you, but she's back to almost a pack a day." Sara Maria handed me Belinda's thick paper chart. It had "Volume 2" written in a black Sharpie on front, and it was fraying in the corner where someone had tried to repair it with Scotch tape. It needed to be scanned into the EMR, but until then, I was stuck with the heavy folder full of paper notes, lab reports, and hospital records.

I took the chart and cleared a place for it on the desk, skimming over Belinda's weight and blood pressure readings. Both were up compared to prior appointments. I found my note from the last visit, two months before: our plans to adjust her blood pressure medicine, my referral for counseling at the Capital Area Mental Health Center.

Despite my reluctance to see her, I did like Belinda. A fifty-eight-year-old white woman with curly gray hair, Belinda had first come to see me two years earlier, after a heart attack. On her good days, Belinda was friendly and funny. We both loved animals, and she often brought in stories about a new rescue cat she couldn't resist keeping or the misadventures of her two Chihuahua mixes. I enjoyed her company and smiled at her flamboyant, flowery dresses. But she was a handful, and recently her depression and other medical problems had eclipsed any "good" in her days. Her blood pressure was uncontrolled, and after promising she would never, ever pick up another cigarette, she had apparently started smoking again. Her visits often took twice as long as our allotted time, leaving me frantic and rushed for the whole session.

Taking a deep breath, I opened the door. "Hi, Belinda. What's going on?"

This was not going to be a quick encounter. She was already in tears, her face red and puffy. I sat down on a stool and steeled myself against an onslaught of impossible problems.

"Charlie can't work," she stammered, referring to her husband. "His boss is threatening to lay him off. . . . He can't lift since he hurt his shoulder." Her husband, also my patient, had been injured three weeks before. He was a kind and steady partner for Belinda. He had helped her through her heart attack and a recent surgery, and he braved his wife's increasingly frequent days of depression. After the injury, I had seen him, ordered x-rays (normal), and told him to rest, which was a joke because he couldn't rest and keep his job as a construction worker.

"Oh, Belinda, I'm so sorry. That's probably part of the reason your blood pressure is so high today," I said, sympathetic to Charlie's plight but trying to focus the visit on her.

"I stopped that one medicine—that little white pill. The pharmacy tried to charge me thirty dollars when I went to pick it up last time. Usually it's only five dollars." Tears began to trickle down her cheeks again.

"That's probably the hydrochlorothiazide—the one that makes you pee a lot?"

She nodded.

"Well, at least we have an explanation for your pressure."

Finances were tight. I knew that, and her mother-in-law was in the hospital again. Belinda had failed to complete the lab tests that I had ordered at her last visit, and I had no idea why the pharmacy was suddenly charging more for the same medicine. Meanwhile, I could hear my next patient, Mandy, through the wall as she was going through the intake process with the medical assistant. Mandy was a classic vampire—my term for those life-sucking patients whose ceaseless demands and negativity left me depleted and exhausted. Her angry voice was unmistakable.

One thing at a time. I'm with Belinda now.

"Have you had any recent chest pain or shortness of breath?" I asked.

"Well, I always have some shortness of breath. . . ."

"No chest pain?"

She shook her head. I patted the white paper covering the exam table, indicating that I wanted to start the exam, and she slowly climbed up onto the table.

Her curly hair reeked of smoke. I suppressed a cough as I listened to her heart and lungs through her red and purple dress. She sounded fine, but most people do. With occasional exceptions, the physical exam is far less important than the patient history for gathering important information. I sometimes listened to a patient's heart and lungs just so I could check off the box in the chart. I had also noticed that patients will often comment that a doctor "didn't do anything" if the physical exam is left out, even if the doctor spent thirty minutes discussing a patient's depression.

"Okay, well, your heart and lungs sound good, but I'm concerned about the smoking."

She looked away. "I know. . . ."

"What do you think about trying that Wellbutrin we talked about last time? It might help both with quitting smoking and with the depression. It seems like maybe the Prozac alone isn't doing the trick."

"I don't know," she said. "I'm already on so many medicines."

I regretted that I didn't have more time for a lengthy discussion about depression, smoking, anything. I needed to get moving to the next room. I could hear my next patient's loud voice through the wall again. I couldn't make out all her words, but by the frequent pauses, I figured she was on her cell phone. I caught the gist of it: ". . . So I said, 'What's it gonna be, asshole: me or the dog?'"

"Okay. I'm going to give you a new prescription for the blood pressure medicine that the pharmacy overcharged you for. Try different pharmacies. I know this medicine is on the four-dollar list at Walmart. You shouldn't have to pay more than that." I paused. I didn't want her to feel rushed even if I did.

"Okay," she said.

"I'm also going to give you some information on the Wellbutrin and a depression questionnaire for you to fill out before you come back to see me," I said.

She nodded as I handed her the questionnaire. I suggested a follow-up appointment in two weeks and reminded her about the need for blood work beforehand. She agreed.

"Please tell Charlie I hope he feels better. I know this is a hard time for y'all," I said, opening the door. "I'll see you in two weeks."

I was finished with her sooner than I'd predicted, but I didn't feel like we'd accomplished much. Even so, I was already fifteen minutes behind schedule. (I know patients hate it when their doctor runs late. What they probably don't realize is that we hate it more.) I typed a quick note summarizing our visit and saw the next patient, who regaled me with the whole story of her boyfriend's terrifying pit bull. Then I rushed into two more rooms to adjust one man's heart failure medicines and talk to another patient about chronic back and knee pain. Then I went in to see Ms. Morris.

Ms. Morris was an elderly woman with multiple medical problems, including dementia, diabetes, and high blood pressure. She was blind and, as best I could tell, spent most of her days sitting in a chair, listening to soap operas. It must have been a lonely existence.

She usually came in with a family member, though today she had a home health assistant who was busy with something on her phone. Her blood pressure was thirty points too high, as usual, but she was completely unconcerned about it. She was focused on a rash on her legs and trunk.

"Hi, Ms. Morris," I said, touching her hand and for some reason speaking louder than usual, as if that would help compensate for the fact that she couldn't see me. I nodded to the assistant who barely glanced at me.

"Doc, I've got this rash, and it just keeps on itchin' and itchin.' My daughter gave me two kinds of cream, but that just makes it worse."

"Well, that sounds pretty frustrating," I said. "Let's take a look. Where is it bothering you the most?" I wanted to move things along so that we could talk about her blood pressure and abnormal lab results, but I knew she wouldn't pay any attention to my concerns if I didn't listen to hers first. Fair enough.

"It's all over. It's a bad one." Ms. Morris lifted the edge of her worn yellow dress. I could see a few red bumps on her legs, but mostly I saw excoriations—linear marks from her scratching. I examined her abdomen and chest. Her mid back was clear, but all the areas she could reach were covered in scratch marks.

"Have you used any new detergents or soaps?" I asked, looking directly at the assistant, who shook her head while continuing to stare at her phone.

"I think it's them bugs from the cat," Ms. Morris said.

"You mean fleas? Do you have a cat with fleas?"

"My granddaughter's cat . . ."

The home health aide interrupted. "They have three cats, and they all have fleas. She doesn't want us to do anything about it."

"They don't have fleas," said Ms. Morris.

"I thought you said the cats had bugs that were causing your rash," I said.

"It's that big pill that's causing them bumps," said Ms. Morris, rocking slowly as she talked. "I can't swallow it, and I have to chew it. It makes me sick."

I sighed, quietly. At least she couldn't see me roll my eyes.

"Okay, well the name of that big pill is metformin, and you've been taking it for your diabetes. But your labs indicate that your kidney function is getting worse, so we're going to have to stop it." I paused.

"Oh," she said, reaching to scratch her leg with long, rough fingernails.

"I'm going to want your family to increase the amount of insulin they're giving you, and you all really need to get rid of the fleas." I again was making a recommendation that I knew my patient was unlikely to follow. "I'm going to write down some instructions for your daughters, and I'm going to send in a prescription for a medicine that can help with the itching. But that medicine may make you tired. Is that okay?"

"Them bumps is keeping me up. I can't sleep," she said.

"Well, I understand that. This medicine should help with both problems," I said. I leaned toward the home health aide and waved my hand a little so that she finally looked up. "Can you make sure someone cuts her fingernails?" The aide agreed, though I had little confidence it would happen.

"Look, Ms. Morris, I share your concern about the rash, but I am even more concerned about your blood pressure," I said, opening her paper chart and reviewing her blood pressure readings from the last several visits: twenty to thirty points high every time, despite medicine additions and adjustments. "Are you taking the medicines I've prescribed for you?"

She didn't say anything but scratched her leg again.

"She doesn't like to take her medicine," the aide said.

"I already drink too many pills," she said, turning in the general direction of her home health aide. "What happened to my soda?"

"You finished it in the car on the way here," her aide said.

"Oh."

"Look, I am very worried that you are going to have a stroke or a heart attack if we can't get your blood pressure down. I think this may also explain why your kidney function is getting worse."

"Can you get me some kind of cream for this rash? I can't sleep worth nothing!"

"Okay. I'm going to write down the name of a cream your daughters can buy for you without a prescription. And I'm going to increase your insulin, stop your metformin, and add a new medicine for your high blood pressure." I made a quick note for the home health aide, suggesting hydrocortisone for the rash, and explained that I'd send the other prescriptions to the pharmacy electronically. "Can you make sure she gets the new prescriptions?" I asked the aide.

She held up a finger, indicating I should wait for a second, clicked some buttons on her phone, and then nodded.

"I need to see you back in a month to recheck some labs and your blood pressure. Also, please take the medicines I've given you, especially your insulin and the ones for your blood pressure."

"This rash is driving me crazy."

"I know. I hope it gets better," I said, opening the door of the room, taking a deep breath, and shutting the door before she could say anything else.

I spent the next ten minutes writing instructions for Ms. Morris and her family and then finishing my note in her chart. I was impatient with her for not understanding the seriousness of her health conditions, for not following instructions. I was frustrated with myself, too, for being impatient. Ms. Morris had barely more than an elementary school education. She was also African American and low income. She had undoubtedly faced discrimination and struggles that

I could only imagine. And she had dementia and was blind. What did I expect?

By then, I was thirty minutes behind.

I wondered for the millionth time how other doctors could see thirty, forty patients in a day. I was exhausted after five. I had an inferiority complex about my efficiency and patient productivity that I couldn't shake. I berated myself daily for my inability to speed up, for my need to look up medication dosages, to remind myself of new treatment options for eczema or osteoporosis. I told myself that I needed to sharpen my skills, learn to interrupt politely, address the main problem, and exit the room. I read articles about how to "work smarter, not harder," "13 Ways to Be More Efficient." But I was slow. I couldn't seem to change that or make peace with it. And now I had to tell Sherry that she had diabetes.

"Hi, Dr. Doggett," Sherry said as I opened the door. She sat on the exam table, wearing slacks and a gray shirt. She held out her hand.

"Hey, Sherry. It's good to see you again," I said, shaking her hand. "How are you doing?"

"Well, I guess not so great. My blood pressure's up. My migraines aren't any better," she said. "I've been working two jobs. It's just a lot."

"Sounds like it," I said. Two jobs, sometimes more. My patients couldn't get a break. Sherry was middle-aged with a couple of teenagers at home if I remembered correctly. Now I was about to make things even more difficult. It sucked, and I didn't know exactly how to break the news.

"I'm glad you were able to come in today because we need to talk about your labs," I continued. "Your blood pressure is up, and I think we need to treat that, but I'm also concerned because it looks like you have diabetes."

"You know, I had a feeling about that," she said.

"Well, it's not too unusual to see it in families. I think you said your mom has it?"

"Yeah . . ." Sherry looked away. "She did have it. She passed a few months ago."

"Oh, I didn't realize that. I'm sorry."

"My brother has it, too. He's not as bad as my mom, but both of them had to take insulin. My mom also had problems with her feet. Nerve damage or something."

"Yeah. Neuropathy, nerve damage," I said, nodding. "Diabetes is hard to avoid sometimes with that kind of family history. But the good news is that your other labs are normal, and at least we caught it before it caused more problems for you."

I was glad we had found Sherry's diabetes, that she had come to see me and gotten her lab tests. Her diagnosis wasn't a surprise. As a Black woman, Sherry faced nearly twice the risk of diabetes as a white person, and her family history compounded her odds further. Still, over 20 percent of people with diabetes—the seventh leading cause of death in the United States—don't know they have it.[1] I was on a mission to make sure none of those 20 percent were among my patients.

"I don't want to go on insulin," Sherry said.

"You don't have to now. You may need to at some point in the future, but not yet." I went on to explain that diet and exercise were the most important treatments for early diabetes, though I also planned to write a prescription for an oral diabetes medication, metformin—the same medicine I'd just stopped for Ms. Morris.

"I know I need to lose weight," Sherry said. "It's just so hard to find the time to exercise. And I don't have time to cook. . . ." She took a deep breath. "But I don't want to end up like my mom."

"It sounds like you have a lot going on," I said. "I know it's hard to hear this news on top of everything else."

I wanted time to process this new diagnosis with Sherry. It was a big deal to have diabetes—a life-changing chronic disease. She was stoic, but how did she really feel? I also wanted to do diet planning, to map out an exercise routine that could sync up with her work schedule, to talk to her about proper diabetic footcare. I wished I at least had someone to refer her to—a diabetes educator or dietician—to provide more guidance and support. But I could only write her prescriptions and move on.

I had to fit in an unscheduled patient, Javier, for a flare of his gout, and then I saw Cassandra for her well-woman exam. When my final patient showed up with an upper respiratory infection and *nothing else wrong*, I could hardly believe it. Small favors.

Even after my last patient was dismissed, though, I wasn't really done. Returning to my office, I again saw the piles of papers awaiting my attention. I wanted to turn around and walk out again. For a moment, I fantasized. *What if I ignored those orders for home health, the x-ray reports, the messages from the pharmacy asking for refill authorizations? What if I just got in my car and drove back to the lake? Would it really matter?* I could never be enough for my patients, who needed so much. So many days I felt useless, unable to help anyone. But I willed myself to sit down at my desk, to pick up the first message.

CHAPTER 5

Striving for Perfection

October 2009

I had to be *that* mom, the one who always makes a homemade birthday cake, even if that meant thumping out the cake from the pan at 11:00 PM. This year, I also had to attend the Halloween festival at my daughters' preschool, even if that meant rushing through an afternoon of patient care and still arriving late. Then there was Jess's pumpkin-carving party, a jog the next morning at the lake with Ella and Clara in the double jogger, a family brunch, Clara's second birthday party, and trick-or-treating. The weekend was as packed as an overstuffed suitcase because I didn't want to miss a thing. I was greedy that way.

The cake, of course, needed pumpkin orange icing. The store didn't sell orange icing or even orange food coloring, so in the tiny window between brunch and party, I leaned on the kitchen counter and mixed red and yellow to get just the right hue. Don, now a hospital-based pediatrician, came home from his day shift, armed with pizza and balloons. I barely glanced at him.

As I hopscotched through the weekend, I scolded myself about striving for perfection and my tendency to focus on deficiencies. The metaphorical glass, to me, was not only half empty. If even one sip had been taken, I focused on the missing sip.

A lopsided cake or the wrong color icing was hardly a big deal. My obsession to fill every moment and get everything just right meant I was harried and impatient. It was baseline behavior, I guess. I couldn't watch a movie without working on a scrapbook or folding laundry. During conference calls even now, I make granola or do sit-ups. I'm not sure if it's habit or character, but it's "me," that's for sure. My internal drill sergeant never let me rest: Do more. Try harder. One more mile. Ten more push-ups. Perfect orange icing.

Monday morning came, and I was happy to be done with the weekend. But something wasn't right. I couldn't quite put my finger on it—the feeling that came over me—but I struggled to get out of bed. I still managed my morning run, but it was slow and labored, not the invigorating start to the day I had imagined. A peculiar cloudiness hung over me.

"How are you doing?" my handsome husband asked as I walked through the door. He was pouring milk into a bowl of Cinnamon Life cereal. The coffee maker gurgled, and NPR hummed along with the morning news: The Yankees were one game short of a World Series victory. An Afghan presidential candidate had just dropped out of the race. Scientists had decoded the DNA of a pig.

"I'm not great. I feel kind of off, kinda dizzy."

"Dizzy?" Don repeated.

"I think that's the best way to describe it. And I slept like ten and a half hours last night," I said, wiping my forehead with a dish towel. "Maybe I'm getting sick."

"You still went running though? Was that a good idea?"

"Maybe . . . I don't know. I thought it might help. But no. If anything, I feel worse."

Don knew about the drill sergeant. I couldn't miss my morning run.

"Feel better," he said, rubbing my shoulder, before grabbing his backpack. "I'm headed to the hospital."

"Okay." I stood up and headed upstairs to awaken the kids.

I tried to ignore the dizziness as I saw patients that morning. Perhaps some new symptoms would pop up, clues to my mystery illness. A sore throat? Earache? Congestion? Fever? But no respiratory virus declared itself. I couldn't think about it, though. I had more urgent concerns.

Marvin was back, struggling with a heart failure exacerbation. His pale legs were swollen, and his breathing was labored and rapid. Dementia and schizophrenia limited his ability to give me a decent history, and he was disheveled, his long gray hair unwashed and at least two buttons missing from his shirt.

"How are you, Marvin?" I asked, glancing up from the chart.

"Fine," he said. Funny the number of sick people who waded through my office, only to tell me they were "fine."

"You look like you're having a little trouble with your breathing today," I said. "And your blood pressure's really high. Did you miss any medicine?"

"I don't think so," he said.

After listening to his lungs, I called his home health nurse to get the full story. Like Ms. Morris, the older woman with the rash, Marvin had both Medicare and Medicaid, government insurance programs that provided far better support than my uninsured patients ever received.

I loved Marvin's nurse. We had never met in person, but several years of phone calls had left us well acquainted. Marvin had followed me to the new clinic from the last place I worked, and his nurse and I shared a fondness for this strange and quiet man. We had each other's cell phone numbers, and I could always count on her to answer. She had practically adopted Marvin and would check on him even on her days off. But despite her help, he struggled.

"I'm glad he showed up today," she said.

"Me too. Unfortunately, I think he's volume overloaded," I said. "And his pressure's 174/100. I just rechecked it myself."

Marvin's uncontrolled blood pressure was increasing his heart's workload. Because his heart couldn't pump effectively, blood got backed up into his lungs, making it difficult to breathe. He would never complain to me, but I could tell he was having a hard time.

"I'm not surprised," his nurse said. "He was out of his diuretic and lisinopril last week. He said he'd pick it up, but I don't think he did. I'll go get it this afternoon." Marvin's seventy-six-year-old girlfriend was in the hospital, and he didn't have anyone at home to look after him.

"I'll give him a dose of both of those meds now," I said. "Can you check on him this evening? I think he'll be okay once he gets some of the fluid off."

We then discussed a way to get his cardiology appointment re-scheduled and his cholesterol medicine refilled. I went back to share the plan with Marvin, though I knew he would forget as soon as he left.

All morning, I tried to maintain a steady pace. I continued to chalk up my dizziness to a virus and tried to put it out of my mind. I wanted to just quit and collapse into bed, but I plowed through my patient visits and tasks, trying to accomplish as much as possible before my symptoms got worse. I managed, at last, to track down someone to help with Faith's outrageous radiology bill. I even let myself imagine that I might get a lunch break, but then Sara Maria handed me the chart for my last patient, a new one. "She's pretty upset," she said. "Good luck!"

Best not to think. Just go.

I entered the room to find a petite young woman with short, neon-pink hair pacing the floor. She was dressed in a red leather dress with bright, striped tights and vintage black boots.

"Oh my God! I have these headaches that won't quit!" she blurted out before I could ask what was wrong. "My sister says they're migraines, but I don't think so. I mean, aren't migraines supposed to go away? These headaches never go away, and I can't sleep. I haven't slept in, like, two weeks."

Amber was hyped up, and her anxiety was so contagious that I had to consciously take deep breaths to relax myself while I was in the room with her.

"I've taken like a hundred Tylenol and Advil, and nothing helps. And now I'm going to be kicked out of my apartment because my roommate can't stand me being up all night, and my sister will only let me stay with her for, like, four or five days. I'm gonna be a bag lady," she continued, waving her hands, wiping away angry tears as she paced the room.

I interrupted her. "Okay, Amber. I'm glad you're here. I can tell you've got a lot going on. Let's start by taking a deep breath, and then let's figure out how I can help."

"I can't sit still. I think I'm going crazy!" she said.

"You don't have to sit down, but take a couple deep breaths with me." I needed them almost as much as she did.

She stood still for the first time, leaning on the exam table and breathing deeply.

"So, I'm hearing that you're having problems with terrible headaches and with sleep," I said.

"And I think I'm going to get fired today, but that's just as well, 'cause I can't stand those people anyway. My boss is the biggest asshole. I came in like two minutes late yesterday, and he—"

I jumped in again. "Whoa! Okay, okay," I said, trying to slow things down. "You do have a lot of stress right now. Let's back up and try to take this one thing at a time. Tell me more about the headaches."

She ran her hands through her pink hair and surprised me by finally sitting down. I was relieved that she was my last patient, that I didn't have anyone else waiting for me. Someone like Amber couldn't be limited to a fifteen-minute visit. *But why did she have to pick today of all days?* My mind felt cloudy, slow. This was too much.

I managed to piece together a complicated history that was not atypical of the many young adult patients I'd seen in clinics over the years. The classic story goes something like this: After a rough childhood, a kid leaves home and tries to make a go of it on her own but then loses a job, breaks up with a partner, or gets hooked on drugs and ends up lost in a downward spiral. In Amber's case, she and her sister, who seemed to be her primary support person, had come to Austin the year before from Oklahoma. Her sister, who was a couple of years older, had found a semi steady job cutting hair. Amber had enrolled in classes at the community college but then dropped out. She now was living with a roommate she hated and working at a laundromat, with an occasional gig as a stripper at a downtown bar. Her various symptoms—headaches, insomnia, aches, and pains—had been exacerbated by her job and unstable living situation. Her all-consuming nervous energy limited her ability to work, think, sleep, and plan.

I thought of the Mood Disorder Questionnaire (MDQ) I sometimes gave patients to screen for bipolar disorder:

Has there ever been a period of time when you were not your usual self and . . .

. . . you were so irritable that you shouted at people or started fights or arguments?

. . . you got much less sleep than usual and found you didn't really miss it?

. . . you were much more talkative or spoke faster than usual?

. . . thoughts raced through your head or you couldn't slow your mind down?

. . . you were so easily distracted by things around you that you had trouble concentrating or staying on track?

. . . you had much more energy than usual?[1]

Yes, yes, and yes. I didn't need the questionnaire. Bipolar disorder, otherwise known as manic depression, is both common and unruly. Affecting an estimated 2.6 percent of the U.S. population, the condition often reveals itself during young adulthood.[2] Depressive episodes can be dark and incapacitating. Rates of suicide may be as high as 19 percent among people with bipolar disorder—ten to thirty times greater than in the general population. For every completed suicide, many more attempts are made.[3] During manic episodes, patients are often extremely short-tempered, anxious, and impulsive. Back in medical school, I abruptly decided not to become a psychiatrist when, during a routine intake interview in the emergency room, a manic patient advanced toward me and screamed, "I could kill you right now!"

Her unprovoked fury left me shaking and terrified. I believed her and, trying to look calm and intentional, stood up and fled the room.

Amber's mania didn't appear to be characterized by violent thoughts or actions, but it was still dangerous and disabling. I tuned out her continued barrage of grievances and planned what to do next. She needed psychiatric care, but even for insured patients, mental health services were limited. I was uncomfortable treating her on my own, and the psychiatric emergency room was probably the only way I could get her the urgent help she needed. But I wasn't sure I could convince her to go.

". . . And I swear the only time I slept in the last month was when I took my roommate's Xanax and Ambien. I think I need my own prescription for Xanax," she continued.

Kim tapped on the door. I cracked it open.

"Dr. Doggett, you've got a phone call," she said.

"I'm sorry—I better get this. I'll be right back," I said to Amber as I exited to the hallway.

Thank God.

"Is this a real phone call or a 'phone call'?" I said, using air quotes.

"No, I just knew that you had been in there awhile, and Terri needs your help with another patient," she said. "What can I do?"

We ducked into Kim's tiny office that she had created from a storage closet. The room was so packed we barely had room to stand. Stacks of charts cluttered her desk, almost burying the monster bobble head from *Where the Wild Things Are*—a gift from Terri—and the shoulder rest she used to position her phone during long calls with patients. Her white coffee mug with a silver snowflake sat precariously near the edge. I smiled at her old badge, with a picture that made her look like a goblin. The staff had nicknamed her "Gobby" when they saw the photo, and Kim, attractive and able to make fun of herself, fully embraced the joke. We stood whispering since the walls of the clinic were as soundproof as cardboard.

"This girl is manic and needs to see a psychiatrist—she needed one like two months ago, actually," I said, wishing I knew a psychiatrist who could see her in their office but knowing that would never happen. "The only way to get her on the list for mental health services will be through the psych ER, but I think she's going to pitch a fit."

"I'm on it," she said. "Terri's in the first exam room. I think she wanted you to see that kid's rash. I'll go talk to Amber."

Finding urgent psychiatric care for someone without insurance was a near impossibility in most of Texas. A shortage of psychiatrists combined with low reimbursement rates, prior authorization hassles, and various restrictions on medications and numbers of visits had created a mental health crisis. Even for insured people, psychiatrists were limited and often expensive; many charged patients directly to avoid dealing with insurance companies. The situation hasn't improved. A 2022 report by Mental Health America ranked Texas fifty-first among states and Washington, DC, in access to mental health care.[4]

Lamenting my lack of better options for psychiatric treatment and the limitations of my own scope of practice and experience, I returned with Kim to the exam room where Amber was sitting down, remarkably, and fiddling with her phone. She glanced up.

"Amber, I can't give you a prescription for Xanax. It's very addictive and can be dangerous, but I do think you need some help." She tried to interrupt, but I held my ground. "I think you're having trouble with sleep and anxiety because of a condition called bipolar disorder. You need to see a psychiatrist and start medication."

Kim jumped in. "I'd like to just talk with you for a couple minutes so we can figure out how to get you more help. It won't take long."

"I'll be back soon," I said. "I'm going to see someone else who's been waiting awhile, and then I'll check back in with you. Promise."

Kim had a knack for handling patients like Amber. Not only could she defuse a tense situation, but she could be persuasive in convincing patients to take their medicine or, as in this case, get to the psychiatric ER for urgent care that was beyond the scope of our clinic. When I returned to the room, after helping Terri with a little boy whose fungal rash had turned into an infection warranting antibiotics, Kim was handing Amber a map.

"So, she's going to go right now to the psych ER, and then she's going to call to let us know how it went," Kim explained. "I've given her a follow-up appointment here next week so that we can make sure she's getting the help she needs."

"Okay, great," I said, relieved. "Amber, I'm really glad you came in today. It sounds like you've really been dealing with a lot, and I think we can help you get this sorted out, but it's important now that we get you psychiatric care."

She looked at Kim. "Thanks. I'll go right now."

I ate lunch while driving to an afternoon meeting where we talked about productivity expectations for the clinic, future funding, and foundation support. The discussion left me more dizzy—and demoralized—than before. The clinic was barely sustainable, yet I was being asked to see more patients, more quickly, while maintaining quality. It was an impossible task.

The same double bind plagued community clinics like mine and private practices all over the country. In medical school we were taught to be thorough, to be present, and to really listen to our patients. Ask open-ended questions. Get a past medical history, a social history, a family history, an occupational history. Do a complete review of systems to cover ailments of every body part. Don't skimp on the physical exam. Consider all diagnostic possibilities. Don't miss anything.

Once training was complete, we learned the real goal: see as many patients as you can, as fast as you can, while not getting sued. During medical school, our professors lectured on the stages of mitosis and the Krebs cycle, but our curriculum lacked training on budgets, office management, and navigating the health care bureaucracy. Now, each time I attended a meeting, I felt like I was learning a new language while being prodded to move faster, do more, hurry up. But I couldn't do more. Even on a good day, when I was clearheaded and well rested, I couldn't see Marvin and Amber and all the others in fifteen-minute increments, wrapping up the visits with nice, tidy notes. I couldn't speed up or I would miss something. All I could do was admit defeat.

CHAPTER 6:

Something Bad

November 2009

As a physician, I'm adept at matching symptoms with a cause. It's a useful skill, one that's saved my family many trips to the doctor for sore throats, allergies, and ankle sprains. The downside is paranoia. In medical school we learn to think of the worst possible diagnoses every time we see a patient to make sure we don't miss Something Bad. Chest pain could be heart disease or a serious blood clot in the lungs. Joint pain could be rheumatoid arthritis. A cough could mean lung cancer or tuberculosis. Fever and fatigue, without a clear source, could be leukemia. And dizziness? Well, it could be an inner ear infection, anxiety, stress, sleep deprivation, a virus . . . but there's always the possibility of a brain tumor.

The week wore on, and still my symptoms didn't improve. The dizziness was constant and steady, but it didn't turn into anything else like a cold or an ear infection. It wasn't vertigo or room-spinning dizziness or motion sickness. The sensation—an unpleasant buzz combined with something akin to jet lag—lingered like a patient who had just "one more thing" to discuss long after the visit should have ended. It made me volatile and frustrated. I could drive. I could work. I could see patients. But everything was harder, and nothing made it go away. I couldn't summon the patience to read "one more story" to Ella and Clara at bedtime. I didn't want to talk to Kim about a possible clinic remodel to create more space, to give her a real office. Hell, I didn't have the energy to put gas in my car.

After several days, when I started noticing double vision along with the dizziness, that brain-tumor thought—unwelcome, but persistent—crept into my mind. *Don't be ridiculous*, I told myself. *There's no way I have a brain tumor. Get real.*

But I didn't know what else could explain my symptoms.

Doctors know lots of other doctors. We call one another for free advice: choosing the right medicine for a patient or developing a treatment plan. In my clinic I often contacted other physicians to ask for favors. I talked to friends and colleagues to solve diagnostic dilemmas and explore next steps in a medical workup.

This time, I was the medical mystery. I kept racking my brain for an explanation and willing myself to make it disappear. I didn't want to ask another busy doctor for help, to inconvenience someone and steal precious minutes from her day. But I needed to understand what was happening and when it would stop. I had seen patients who delayed care out of fear, and it never turned out well. I was scared, but for me, the not-knowing was worse than anything. I called a neurologist acquaintance on her cell.

"I'm so sorry to bother you. Do you have a second?"

"Of course," she said. "It's no bother."

I reviewed my symptoms with the doctor. She listened and asked a few questions: Had this happened before? Did I have anything else wrong? Did I have any other medical problems? No, nothing.

"Can you stop by at lunch?" she asked.

"Are you sure? I don't want to take your lunch hour," I said, struck by the incredible gift this woman was offering: a same-day consultation with an expert.

"It's no problem," she said. "It's been a slow morning."

An hour later, I logged off my computer, mumbled an excuse to Terri and Kim, and got in my car, grateful that my morning had been slow as well.

The neurologist did a quick exam, looking in my eyes, checking my cranial nerves, evaluating my strength, sensation, and reflexes. She tested my gait and ability to walk heel-to-toe. I passed. I could move both eyes, arms, and legs normally. I could stick out my tongue and move it from side to side. I could stand still with my eyes closed and not stumble or fall. I could touch her finger and then my nose, going back and forth without difficulty. Normal. Everything was normal.

So why did I feel like shit?

"You know, it's pretty rare to have something really serious and a totally normal exam," she said. "I think you're going to be okay. Maybe this dizziness is some sort of atypical migraine?"

I'd never had a migraine. This explanation didn't seem likely, but it fit as well as anything. Common things are common, we're taught in medical school. If you hear hoofbeats, it's probably a horse, not a zebra.

"It seems like a weird migraine, but you would know better than me," I said, pulling out my car keys. "Can't I give you my insurance information? And I'm glad to pay the co-pay . . ."

"No need," she interrupted. "Keep in touch. We can reconnect if you're not getting better."

Somewhat reassured—and still thanking my lucky stars for being able to see the doctor—I went to buy meclizine, a medicine commonly used for dizziness. I took one pill before returning to the clinic, waited, and was underwhelmed with its effect. The next day I tried Advil and Sudafed. Maybe they helped? The placebo effect is powerful—nearly 40 percent of people will feel better with a sugar pill.[1] In some instances, people will feel better even when they know they are getting a placebo.[2] My eagerness to feel better made me susceptible to the placebo effect, but my awareness of its power made me second-guess any perceived benefit.

I was desperate. Each morning, I would awaken and, for a second, feel normal. My head would be clear, and I'd feel a rush of motivation and excitement about the day. Was the dizziness gone? If only. It was there, waiting for me to fully wake up so it could wrap me in a debilitating fog. When would it end? I *needed* to know.

It reminded me of the countless conversations I'd had with Don about the importance of a bedtime for the kids. "Look, Don," I'd say. "I know you want to have some flexibility and not feel rushed when you read Ella a bedtime story, but I need to have an endpoint. I need for them to have a bedtime even more than *they* need to have a bedtime."

After a few more days of symptoms, I was getting pissed off. I wanted to jump out of the cloud that had trapped me, that compounded the challenges of patient care and parenthood, but nothing seemed to make a difference.

Don worked several evenings that week, leaving me alone with the kids. It wasn't his fault or his choice. As a fellow physician, I knew that as well as anyone. The hospital didn't operate only during normal business hours. The schedule was set well in advance, and he couldn't easily change or drop a shift.

But I still didn't like it. Alone with the kids, I felt like each task—dinner, baths, bedtime—was an impossible hurdle. "Can't y'all just get ready for bed by yourselves?" I wanted to shout.

At one point, I did ask Ella to help. "Sweetie, can you please run back downstairs to get Clara's toothbrush? I guess we left it down there this morning. I'm feeling a little sick."

"No!" she declared. "I don't want to go downstairs."

I blinked back tears and stomped down the stairs, reminding myself that she was only four years old.

My feeling of bitterness over our uneven division of kid-related labor was more acute than ever. "Why don't you get more help from a sitter?" Don would ask when I lamented my lack of free time. *You.* Not *we.* Typical.

I felt a deep-rooted obligation to be there for the kids when I wasn't working. And we did have fun, creating forts with blankets and sofa cushions or building skyscrapers or an airport with blocks. Ella and I loved reading classic children's books: the original *Wizard of Oz,* the complete collection of Beatrix Potter. Clara kept us laughing with her wild dress-up games, colorful outfits paired with silly hats and sunglasses. I just couldn't turn the kids over to someone else. But now I was sick and overwhelmed, and I didn't have a backup plan for getting extra support.

Don's help was sporadic, about as reliable as finding a parking space in downtown Austin. His variable work hours meant we couldn't settle on a routine. One week he might take on the laborious task of putting Clara to bed every night, but the next week, he might work three evenings. My predictable schedule, greater availability, and aptitude for planning meant that I was the Default Parent—the kids came to me first for everything, night or day. I was the CEO, the conductor, but also the worker bee. Don played his part when he could and, well, when he felt like it. Eight years into our marriage we had established our roles, but I never stopped resenting my appointment as Household Manager and his as the Occasional Assistant.

I was in good company. Two decades of research by the Bureau of Labor Statistics showed that working women covered nearly two-thirds of childcare responsibilities while their male partners picked up the other third.[3] Don and I agreed, in theory, such a division was unfair. We were closer to 50/50 than the average couple, but the studies validated my reality: I was chief cook and bottle washer. As far as our marriage was concerned, reaching true equality was only a priority for one of us.

At the end of the week, we finally had a family dinner together. "Don, what's going on with me? I still feel like crap, and my vision is all screwed up," I lamented as we were sitting down at the kitchen table. Don was smart—exceptionally so—and I wanted him to make sense of my symptoms. He would know if something was wrong, right?

"I'm sure you're fine," my husband responded as he scooped up pasta and salad. It was our fallback meal—easy to make, acceptable to the kids, and vegetarian. As he handed full plates to Ella and Clara, I marveled at his lack of concern. I might as well have said I'd forgotten to pick up apples. He was used to my freak-outs. Every time I got sick with the slightest thing, I panicked that it must be the worst possible diagnosis. To Don, this time was no different.

I wanted to believe him. "I just don't get why this isn't getting any better," I said.

"You know you always do this."

"I don't always *do this*."

Don and I were good together. We loved dogs and *Seinfeld* and M. Scott Peck's *The Road Less Traveled*. We enjoyed rock concerts and the political skits on *Saturday Night Live*, and we went to movies every chance we got. We agreed that making the bed was a waste of time, but doing laundry and washing dishes were prudent. Don had helped me through college and those long years of medical training. Since he was a year ahead, he was able to tutor me in biochemistry, encourage me to just get through the basic science classes because clinical rotations were much better. During residency Don traveled with me to rural India, totally out of his comfort zone, where we worked in a tiny hospital located on an elephant preserve—all at my urging. But sympathy—that just wasn't his thing.

"You saw the retina doctor for that eye thing, right?" he continued. "And everything was normal."

Don was referring to my recent complaint of cloudy vision, just a few weeks earlier. Two eye doctors and a battery of tests later, I had received a diagnosis: "dry eyes."

"But that was different, that was like . . . I don't know. It just felt like I had dirty contacts, but I didn't. Now I'm having *double* vision," I said. Double vision, known in doctor-speak as diplopia, was often a sign of a more serious problem. Why wasn't Don getting more freaked out?

"So, can you see someone else?" he asked. "Do you even have a primary care doctor?"

I didn't have a family doctor since most of the time I could manage health issues on my own. Don knew that but was irritated with my anxiety. It was easier and more comfortable for him to dismiss me than to acknowledge I might actually be sick.

"Mommy has a doctor—the doctor that helped when she had me," Ella chimed in.

"No, Honey. Mommy doesn't need that kind of doctor," Don smiled. "She needs a psychiatrist."

c——

A few days later, with the dizziness as persistent as ever, and now with Don's encouragement, I sought advice from another physician friend, a respected family doctor and former colleague.

I described my symptoms over the phone, including the fact that my sense of taste was now changing: my raspberries that morning had tasted like water. Without hesitation, she said, "You need an MRI."

Not what I wanted to hear.

I didn't say it, but I knew that "You need an MRI" was code for "This could be Something Bad." I had wanted reassurance, not confirmation of my fear. But I knew she was right.

"It may not be anything," she said, perhaps sensing my concern. "But you need to find out for sure."

I didn't feel comfortable calling the neurologist back. I didn't want to bother her again after she had said I was probably okay. So my friend gave me her recommendation for an ear, nose, and throat (ENT) specialist who might help with the dizziness. The ENT doctor was also a friend of Don's.

"I should have thought of him," Don said, dialing the specialist's cell phone number.

It was a Sunday afternoon, and we were in the backyard. The kids were playing in the sandbox while I was watering the plants, but I stopped to listen as Don reviewed my story with his friend. He sat at the metal table on our patio with his phone pressed to his ear. I was relieved to hear his side of the conversation as he described my condition. He was taking me seriously. After a brief pause, he stood up and passed me the phone.

"What's going on?" the ENT asked.

"Dizziness, taste changes, diplopia," I said. "I saw two eye doctors for cloudy vision a few weeks ago. They did all kinds of tests and said I was fine. But now more stuff is happening, and I'm starting to kind of panic."

"Have you ever had anything like this before?" he asked.

"No." I sat down on our yellow swing, rocking back and forth.

"Do you have any other medical problems or medications?"

"Nothing," I said. "I've always been healthy."

He asked more questions—in essence, providing a free consult over the phone—and gave me an appointment in his office the next day.

"We'll do some hearing tests, and I'll examine you," he said. "It sounds like we need to get an MRI."

I thanked him and hung up. I didn't want to deal with an MRI, with doctors' appointments, with any of it. But at least I was getting help. I wouldn't be the only one trying to figure out what was wrong.

I glanced at the kids. They had no idea anything was going on. They were covered in sand. Clara had smudges on her face. Apparently, she and Ella had decided the sand would be more interesting combined with water from the hose. Bath time was going to be fun.

I walked over to Don and sat down across the table from him, handing the phone back. I summarized the plan: an appointment the next day, probably an MRI.

"Tomorrow? That's fast," he said.

"I know. It's really unbelievable. First the neurologist, and now this," I said. "My uninsured patients have to wait a year to get into an ENT clinic. A year!"

"I know," he said. "Sometimes it really helps to be a doctor."

And educated and middle-class . . . and white.

While I wanted to be color-blind with my patients—to treat every-one equally—that desire blinded me to some of the injustices facing them. One of my patients, in fact, waited two years to get into the ENT clinic, only to be sent away without a diagnosis or treatment plan. Did her race—African American—contribute to the doctor's dismissive attitude? Studies now show that discrimination in health care is pervasive, impacting an estimated one in five people. Discrimination based on race and ethnicity followed by education and income level are the most common types, according to a 2019 survey.[4]

I took so much for granted. I could draw on connections all over the city for immediate attention from doctors who took me seriously. My patients were stuck at the back of the line if they could even find the line in the first place. I was overwhelmed with gratitude that I could sidestep the queue but equally furious that so many others couldn't get what they needed.

The system was and is unfair and unethical. I was more aware than ever, and I felt guilty for being a part of it.

The next day, at the ENT's office, I was ushered into a soundproof room and given a set of headphones. Don had accompanied me, and he stayed in an adjacent room where he could see me through the glass.

"You're going to hear a series of beeps," the audiologist explained. "Raise your hand when you hear the sound."

The experience reminded me of a high-tech version of the hearing tests administered in my old elementary school: low beeps followed by impossibly high beeps that I couldn't register for a few seconds. But it felt more important and formal inside the special room.

Evidently, I managed to hear all the beeps. The doctor commented on my excellent hearing when we were face-to-face. Then he looked in my ears and throat and did his own neurologic exam—all normal as I'd expected. The Dix-Hallpike maneuver was last, a test used to diagnose benign paroxysmal positional vertigo (BPPV), a common cause of dizziness triggered by dislodged calcium deposits in the inner ear.

"I'm sure you know how this is done," he said. "Go ahead and scoot back on the table so your legs are stretched out in front. Turn your head to the side."

"I don't think it's BPPV," I said, "but I know that would be treatable and not a big deal. That'd be a great diagnosis, actually."

The doctor then asked me to lie all the way down so my head stretched off the end of the table, turned with one ear down. He watched my eyes carefully, looking for nystagmus (funny eye twitching) with the movement.

"Are your symptoms any worse?" he asked.

"Nope. Nothing makes me better or worse. It's just constant," I said.

"Okay," he said. "Let's talk."

I sat up again on the table in front of the ENT doctor and awaited his verdict. I let my legs dangle off the table and rubbed my hands together, trying not to fidget.

"You need an MRI," he said . . . *because this could be Something Bad.* I finished the sentence in my head.

Don, who had been sitting across the room, moved to the exam table to take my hand. We both looked at the doctor for more, for a glimmer of hope or a clue to his thoughts. *Wasn't my exam normal? Did he pick up on something wrong?*

"Everything is normal," he said, "except for some very subtle nystagmus, though not like we'd see with BPPV. It may be nothing, but I'm not sure."

Nystagmus? What's that about? And "not sure"? While I appreciated his honesty, I didn't like the sound of that.

I've had to tell many patients over the years that I'm not sure what's going on. "I don't know why your feet hurt when you're driving," or "I'm not sure why your head feels hot while the rest of you is cold." It's always frustrating—for them and for me. Now the uncertainty was personal and alarming, but I didn't want the MRI to provide an explanation. An answer that came from the MRI would mean a problem with my brain. The thought that I *could* have a brain tumor began to morph into a near certainty that I *did* have a brain tumor.

Don wasn't in a joking mood that night. We were both quiet and unusually polite, adding "please" or "thank you" to every sentence as we went through the dinner ritual. Don made pasta and salad again while I shuffled through the mail, tossing most of it into the recycling bin.

"It's going to be fine," he said.

"Thanks. I hope so," I said as I lifted Clara into the high chair and snapped on her bib.

We sat down. I didn't eat. I scooped salad onto Ella's plate and then my own, staring at the walnuts mixed in with the spinach.

An hour later, while Don was putting the kids to bed, I pulled out *Harrison's Principles of Internal Medicine*, the main reference book in the library of every medical student of my generation, to try to piece together my symptoms in a logical way. The book was so large and heavy that I had to use both arms to carry it, shooing our dog, Mocha, out of the way as I walked to the couch. I sat down and took a deep breath. *What causes dizziness, double vision, and taste changes that isn't a brain tumor?*

"Disorders of the sense of taste are caused by conditions that interfere with the access of the tastant to the receptor cells in the taste bud (transport loss), injure receptor cells (sensory loss), or damage gustatory afferent nerves and central gustatory neural pathways (neural loss)," I read. *What the hell does that mean?*

I looked at maps of neurologic pathways I'd memorized in medical school but hadn't seen since. I got lost in the language: superior cerebellar peduncle, medial longitudinal fasciculus, lateral lemniscus, pontine nuclei. *Did I ever understand this stuff? How did I manage to pass my licensing exams?*

Next, I tried to figure out where my brain tumor could be growing without causing headaches but still triggering this bizarre constellation of other symptoms. The taste center of the brain was nowhere near the visual center. I didn't know where the dizziness was coming from. *Could I have multiple brain tumors? Metastases from a cancer somewhere else?* Nothing made sense.

Don cuddled up with me in bed that night, putting his beloved crossword puzzle on the bedside table and sliding his arm underneath me. "Look, Lisa. It really is going to be okay," he said again, almost tearing up. "We can't jump to conclusions. And no matter what happens, I'll be here. I mean, we just have to take it one step at a time."

His unusual emotion and affection both comforted and scared me. "Thanks. I just want it to go away. I just don't want this to change everything," I whispered.

Fortunately, I didn't have patients scheduled the next day. I stumbled through my charts, answered e-mails, and addressed abnormal labs. As I scanned one person's chart, I thought, *too bad this guy has diabetes, but that's nothing compared to my brain tumor.* I imagined that I might never return to the clinic again. Perhaps the MRI would reveal a dangerous mass requiring emergency surgery that would maim me forever. Perhaps I had cancer, just weeks to live.

I couldn't look at the pictures on my desk of my happy, smiling children. The inescapable reality of parenthood weighed on me now, severe and heavy. I could die. That would be okay for me, maybe. I wouldn't feel anything; I wouldn't have to suffer long. But my children were so young, so vulnerable and needy. They would have to live their whole lives without a mother. How unfair to leave Don alone to raise them. We entered parenthood as partners—imperfect and lopsided, perhaps, but committed to sharing our enormous responsibility. Tragic images emerged: small children in a cemetery, milestone events infused with sadness. If only they were a little older. Their existence made my continuing existence imperative.

c⁓

The MRI machine brought to mind an alarm-testing factory. The earplugs provided before the test now made sense. Invented in the 1970s, magnetic resonance imaging (MRI) relies on powerful magnets to create images far more detailed than traditional x-rays. Blamed, in part, for the rising cost of health care, MRIs are expensive. I rarely ordered them or saw MRI reports because my patients couldn't afford them, but I knew MRI machines to be powerful diagnostic tools for brain pathology. They can locate brain tumors and reveal traumatic brain injury, developmental abnormalities, and stroke. They work without exposing patients to radiation. And they are loud. Really loud.

Z-whurp, Z-whurp. BANG BANG BANG. Dat Dat Dat Dat Dat Dat.

I imagined a maniacal scientist, bounding around a large, window-less room, pushing buttons, and pulling levers on huge machines with blinking lights. He was testing new combinations of sounds: security systems, ambulance sirens, smoke alarms. He barked commands to his minions who raced around adjusting more machines.

The shrieks and loud banging continued for at least forty-five minutes, but my growing anxiety eclipsed all other sensations. My whole life could be transformed by whatever this was.

Logically, though I tried to avoid thinking about it, I always knew that I—that anyone—could get sick. I'd seen it happen in my medical training, in my practice. I thought of Daisy, a young mother of three, who had been kicked out of three emergency rooms without a diagnosis for her back pain. Her cancerous spinal tumor was only discovered after I managed to get her a rare, discounted MRI. And Faith. What had she done to deserve incapacitating asthma? Now it was my turn.

The neuroradiologist greeted us as we walked into his dark room. Don and I were grateful he could meet with us right away—another privilege we enjoyed as fellow physicians. I forced myself to stay rigid, to pretend like this was no big deal, though I was almost trembling. Don stood close with an arm around me. The neuroradiologist pulled up the MRI films on a large computer monitor and started to methodically review them with us.

"There's not a brain tumor," he said, "but there are some white matter changes here." He pointed with his pen. "And here."

So, it is NOT normal. Oh my God! What does he mean by "white matter changes"? What is happening? And how is Don staying so calm? He's acting like this is just another day of hospital rounds.

Despite all this drama about having a brain tumor, I didn't really expect them to find anything. I wanted the neuroradiologist to say, "Everything is perfectly normal, and here is a nice psychiatrist who will help you with your hypochondriasis."

My supersmart husband figured it out right away. "So, it's MS," he said as if he were discussing one of his patients.

MS? That didn't make any sense. I got colds and occasional cuts and bruises but never really sick. MS was a big deal. It just wasn't possible. I was dizzy and confused, but Don had to be wrong.

The neuroradiologist pointed at the white spots that weren't supposed to be there. "Yes. The changes here are suggestive of multiple sclerosis."

Suggestive.

"This one white spot near the right frontal horn pretty much confirms the diagnosis."

Confirms.

What?

Don hugged me to his side. I just stood there, dizzy, frozen, stunned. I couldn't believe this was my MRI we were looking at. I would never be normal again. I was now a sick person. MS was incurable—I knew that much. It just didn't seem possible.

"So, I have multiple sclerosis?" I said, surprised that I could muster a calm tone.

"Yes."

CHAPTER 7:

White Spots

November 2009

Numb with disbelief, I still felt rage pounding on the door. *Was I really just diagnosed with MS? How can this be happening?* I was healthy. I had always been healthy. My medical history was boring. The worst disease I'd ever had in my whole life was mono. I'd had stitches once, after cutting my chin at age five on the sharp edge of my parents' sink. I had surgery on my jaw at age sixteen to correct a dental problem. Nothing else. Not even a broken toe. Boring.

I didn't think I was capable of being shocked anymore. Medical training and years of clinical practice had desensitized me. Patients shared stories about being in prison, about living on the streets. Some had escaped violent homes, abusive partners. Others confessed drug use—or they came to me pleading for unwarranted hydrocodone or anxiety medicine. I learned to listen and stay composed, hiding any surprise. In a human sexuality class in medical school, we were shown a porn movie that took all the most graphic portions of multiple films from different porn "genres" and spliced them together into a ten-minute masterpiece. We sat there in a standard classroom watching a movie that I would have been embarrassed to watch alone—that way, we could respond with a calm nod when our patients mentioned their most unusual exploits. I thought I had seen it all. And yet now, somehow, I had been caught completely off guard and was shaken and terrified by my new reality.

I stared at the fuzzy white spots. A hint of a memory drifted to me: medical residency, another dark room, hushed voices, and an MRI riddled with white spots. The patient was a young white woman, early thirties, previously healthy. The radiologist and the neurologist huddled before the pictures, pointing to the lesions, counting them: seven, eight, nine. An MS diagnosis, a high disease burden, limited treatment options. Devastation. Yet I longed to be in that room, reviewing someone else's films and feeling sad with that requisite professional distance about someone else's bad luck.

Don thanked the radiologist as we turned to leave. My black flats squeaked on the tile floor. Exiting and stepping to the side of the door, Don and I stopped and held each other, silent. The dim hall was empty. In the distance we could hear nurses and other doctors walking through adjacent corridors, talking quietly. The air conditioning rumbled nearby, though it was early November. I wanted to push rewind. I imagined our story playing backward as we stepped back into the room, before the radiologist, but this time he would say something different. He would take it back. He would tell me I was okay.

We didn't stay there long. I've never learned to stand still, and even now I needed to get moving, get out of that hospital. Don and I didn't speak, but we each knew how the other felt. To talk would amplify our fear, would make it real. We held hands and walked together back to the car.

With the answer came the questions: *What does this mean? What can I do? Will I be able to keep my job? Will I be able to drive, to run . . . to take care of my kids?* Even my mind couldn't stand still and was jumping ahead, already needing a plan to deal with this news.

"Alright then," I said as we reached the car. "I'm going to call the neurologist again and tell her about the MRI. I think she can tell me what to do next." Launching into planning mode felt comforting and familiar. Step 1: Call neurologist. I was back in control. *Don't think of anything else. Don't analyze. Don't feel anything.* I pulled my sunglasses out of the car cupholder and searched for her number in my phone. Don opened the door to the driver's seat and picked up his own phone to arrange to take off the rest of the afternoon.

"Oh, damn!" the neurologist said when I shared the news.

"Yeah, this kind of sucks." I was fake calm, an art practiced by doctors and parents alike. I was an expert at fake calm, thank God— without it, I'd totally fall apart. "What should I do now? Isn't there some MS doctor in Austin?"

"Yes, you're thinking of Dr. Reynard. He sees most of the MS patients in town," she said.

I remembered an MS doctor from years before. A man had come to my clinic reporting visual changes and a known MS diagnosis. He had been enrolled in a clinical trial, allowing him access to free medications, but he had dropped out. I had called the MS specialist for help but didn't hang onto the doctor's name. I didn't think I'd need to call him again, certainly not for myself.

The neurologist went on to explain that the MS specialist would start high-dose steroids. "Let me give him a call," she said. "We can get those ordered for you. You should call his office to set up an appointment. He can probably see you in a week or two."

"Yeah, that sounds good," I said, though I wondered how I would ever get through the next "week or two" with so much uncertainty, no definitive treatment, and no plan.

My medical training had taught me next to nothing about MS, a progressive brain disease caused by loss of myelin, the substance that coats nerve cells. Estimates vary, but recent studies show it affects roughly 1 in 300 to 350 adults.[1] Yet I had only seen two or three patients with it during my years of practice. I'd never diagnosed anyone and didn't know the symptoms—other than mobility concerns—or the prognosis.

When I got home that afternoon, I went straight to my computer, ignoring the advice of every physician I knew: beware of Dr. Google. Needing information, I now appreciated from a new perspective the desperate search for understanding, for hope.

Incongruous sunshine spilled in through the windows of my small home office as I scrolled through dozens of websites: cartoons of nerve cells, brains, spinal cords; pictures of MRIs and people with canes or in wheelchairs. I was on a mission, focused, driven to find answers.

I didn't like what I read. "No cure." "Permanent damage or deterioration." "A leading cause of disability in young adults." MS, I learned, had the potential to impact nearly every physical function. And as MS grew more severe, so would the symptoms. In other words, this dizziness, double vision, and overwhelming fear—they were only the beginning.

Recalling my recent visual problems, I was especially troubled to learn that MS could destroy the optic nerve or other parts of the central nervous system responsible for vision. It could cause blindness, partial or full, temporary, or sometimes permanent.

While the relapsing, remitting form of MS is more common, meaning I might get better in the coming weeks, many people who initially improve between exacerbations develop progressive MS, accumulating disability and new symptoms over time. Multiple sclerosis doesn't kill, but it cripples.

In third grade, I had participated in the MS Readathon. Gathered in the school cafeteria, my classmates and I listened as a spokeswoman from an MS charity organization shared stories of lives destroyed by multiple sclerosis. What impressed me more than the stories were the prizes we would win at various fundraising levels, including the $150 grand prize shopping spree at a favorite toy store. I fell for the bribery. I made it my mission to win the shopping spree, reading dozens of books and asking neighbors and relatives to support me. I had to settle for a trophy, but I still remembered the pictures of people with canes and walkers featured in the motivational slideshow. They were so distant from me. I should have appreciated my good health. I should have felt lucky, but the thought that I could someday be one of them never occurred to me.

And, of course, I remembered Mr. Sloane, the patient from medical school whose body was wrecked by MS.

At least I had a diagnosis. I read stories of people who had symptoms typical of MS, but their normal spinal taps and MRIs left them frustrated and confused. Others complained of nonspecific symptoms that could be MS but were told they had chronic fatigue syndrome, fibromyalgia, or depression. Some were left in medical purgatory, unable to start treatment, unable to stop searching for answers. As I later learned, the average MS patient waits months to years after symptom onset to find out she has MS. Thanks to my physician contacts, persistence, and Don's support, my diagnosis took just over a week (or a little less than a month if I counted my earlier visual changes as the starting line).

But I wasn't ready to be grateful.

I took care of myself. I was active, healthy—a prude, even. Despite my obsessive exercise, veggie-laden diet, snobby preference for Whole Foods' organic produce, and self-righteous efforts to model healthy behaviors for my kids and my patients, I now had a disabling brain disease. To be saddled with this diagnosis was unfair, wrong, outrageous. It didn't make sense. Some of the pictures I saw showed people smiling. Smiling? How could they be happy about a diagnosis like MS?

Perusing the web felt like putting hiking boots on blistered feet. Information didn't feel empowering. I was at a loss. When I had clinical questions about a patient, researching the problem reduced my anxiety, providing answers, a path forward. But reading about my own chronic brain disease was way too personal. This was me. This was Clara and Ella's mom, Don's wife, Faith's doctor. All hope drained away as I learned about the possible complications that awaited me. Dizziness wasn't even mentioned as a common symptom of MS on most websites. Instead, typical symptoms included numbness, weakness, fatigue, visual problems, gait disturbance, urinary incontinence, cognitive dysfunction. . . . It was a long list.

More questions jumped out at me. *Would I be stuck with dizziness forever? Could I still work? How long would it take for me to be cognitively impaired and immobile?*

Don came to check on me, caught a glimpse of the gloomy pictures on my computer, and dragged me out of my storm of negativity and pessimism.

"This isn't the time to read about MS," he said.

"But I need to learn more. I need—"

"You got an appointment with Dr. Reynard—next Wednesday, right?" he interrupted. "Let him be your doctor."

He was right. I was going to see one of the best. I should let him do his job. Short of completing a four-year neurology residency, followed by an MS fellowship, years of practice, and probably a PhD, I would never know as much as my expert new doctor.

The front door opened. Clara and Ella hurried in with their sitter. Giggling, the kids raced to my little office, just beyond our living room, where I still sat at my desk. Clara's cheeks were flushed with excitement as she climbed into my lap without waiting to be lifted. The kids were talking at the same time, their voices rushed and eager, competing to be the first to tell me about their afternoon at West Austin Park. I started to smile, then stopped. No more smiles; I had MS. But I took a deep breath and let myself be pulled in by those two animated little girls and their nearly palpable, joyful energy.

"Mommy, we went to the park, and we found a butterfly," Ella said.

"You did? How cool!" I said.

"Mommy, Mommy!" Clara said, raising her voice to talk over Ella. "Look!"

Ella held up the delicate orange and black butterfly for my inspection. I just hugged her and squeezed little Clara against my chest, kissing her blond head that still smelled like the pineapple shampoo we'd used the previous night.

It's going to be okay. We're going to be okay, I told myself. I only wished I believed it.

CHAPTER 8

Where's the Beef?

November 2009

The dizziness was the worst. In the days after my diagnosis, it was persistent, constant. And the endpoint, if there even was one, was elusive. The intravenous steroids didn't help. Every morning I awoke hopeful that the dizziness would be gone, only to be struck with disappointment that this day, too, would be difficult. This day, too, would be like having the color stripped from a vibrant photograph. It was the opposite of rose-colored glasses. It was a sour taste permeating every activity, every interaction. I could take the news of my diagnosis, the uncertainty of my future, but I couldn't deal with the dizziness.

One of the first people I consulted, before I could see my new MS neurologist, was a friend of a friend in Seattle.

"She's an acupuncturist, and she has MS," my friend, a fellow physician, had said when she connected us. "She's been through a lot—can probably, you know, relate to what you're going through."

I gave the acupuncturist a call.

I sat on my front porch, on a cloudy and humid November afternoon, holding my phone to one ear and trying to concentrate on our conversation. I struggled to ignore the woozy feeling in my head, and I hoped this woman, though far away in Seattle, would tell me how to feel better. As we exchanged small talk, I imagined her sitting on the floor of her bungalow, candles and books around her, maybe a meditation cushion, a light rain outside.

"So how long have you been a vegetarian?" she asked, after some preliminary questions about my health history and diet preferences. Her tone was more professional than friendly, but I would give her a chance.

"Seventeen years."

"And how long did you breastfeed your children?"

What does that have to do with anything?

"A year with the first one, sixteen months with the second," I answered.

"Well, there you go!" she said. I could almost see her clapping her hands together, satisfied that she had figured me out. "You're depleted. No meat, no protein, two pregnancies, a busy career, and breastfeeding."

Depleted. That's why I got MS?

She went on to explain that in Chinese medicine, they would say my chi was used up. I needed meat to replenish it.

"So, am I going to have this dizziness forever? What can I do to get rid of it, to feel better now?" I asked, near tears at the thought of giving up my vegetarianism.

"Well, I think I'd go eat a big steak and see how I felt," she said.

I ended our conversation after that. I didn't want to hear anymore. I wanted to blow out the candles I imagined around her. I wanted to step on them and tell her she didn't know what the hell she was talking about. I hung up and sat on the porch, crying for a minute before taking deep breaths and going back in the house.

Could she be right? Being vegetarian was part of my identity. I didn't flaunt it or shame my meat-eating friends when they ordered an entrée that once had parents, but I embraced vegetarianism because of my concern for health, animal welfare, and environmental stewardship. Did I need to compromise my values to heal myself?

c⁓

Walking into Dr. Reynard's office, I braced myself for a waiting room full of the kinds of people I'd seen on the Internet, equipped with assistive devices crafted by creative occupational therapists. Instead, the waiting room was mostly empty. Chairs lined the walls, as if they were expecting a crowd, but the room was occupied by just three people—now five, with Don and me. A gray-haired woman sitting next to a metal walker was reading *People* magazine with Patrick Swayze on the cover. A younger couple sat along one wall, both scrolling through their iPhones. They glanced at the TV when the weather forecast flashed across the screen.

Don helped me with the paperwork. We took the stack to divide and conquer. Insurance information, current symptoms, current medications, allergies, past medical history, family history, social history, patient rights and privacy policy, consent for treatment, consent to allow access to my information. It was all there, and some of it had to be repeated on multiple forms. *Did they really need to know about my thyroid nodule and a cousin's skin cancer?* I wondered. *Were the forms at my clinic so onerous?*

We weren't finished yet when the medical assistant summoned us back to an exam room. While Don completed the forms, I leafed through a couple of brochures about various medications I'd never heard of and read e-mail on my phone. Don tapped his foot on the floor. It felt a little like waiting for a blind date or a job interview. We wanted to make a good impression. And we knew that this new doctor would be our pilot on a long, previously unexpected journey. We wanted to be able to trust him, to share the burden of decision-making, to have a reliable source of information. And I wanted to make sure he wouldn't send me out with orders to eat steak.

A few minutes later, Dr. Reynard knocked and opened the door.

Don and I both looked up. This was it. We were meeting my doctor.

"Hi, I'm Dr. Reynard. Let's talk about what's been going on."

What a relief to finally be here with my new MS doctor! I wondered if my patients ever felt such relief to see me, reassured by my smile and "DR." on my name badge.

Dr. Reynard shook our hands and settled on a stool. I noticed the framed diplomas on the wall behind him. MD, PhD. Good.

I reviewed my symptoms and understanding of the current situation: I had an MRI consistent with MS, continued dizziness, and no help from the IV steroids.

Dr. Reynard let me talk, and then he conducted another neurologic exam, which I already knew would be normal, except for possible nystagmus, those repetitive, uncontrolled movements of the eye. Even with my dizziness, I could pass a neurologic exam, including coordination tests and tandem gait, with no perceptible deficits. After the exam, Dr. Reynard pulled up my MRI films on his computer.

"Well, I'd say there's about an 85 percent chance this is MS," he said, indicating with his pen the white spot on the film that I knew was the area of greatest concern. "You have symptoms and MRI changes that are characteristic."

He went on to explain that the white spots on the MRI indicated areas of disruption of the underlying brain tissue. Their location, in my case, was typical for MS.

"There is good news here, too," he said. "We don't see black holes, which indicate potentially irreversible nerve damage. They correlate with disability."

I appreciated his direct manner. He spoke with the confidence that comes with knowing everything about a subject. But no arrogance, thank goodness. And he spoke at my level, addressing me as both a patient and a colleague in a way that seemed just right.

Don squeezed my hand.

"If I have MS, is there some special diet I need to follow? Like, do I have to eat meat?" I asked.

"Well, you need a healthy diet, sure," he said, "but there isn't one MS diet for everyone. I have a lot of patients who are vegetarians. I don't think you have to eat meat."

What a relief! I could work with this guy.

"So, do we need to do a spinal tap to confirm the diagnosis?" Don asked. We both knew this was a possibility. A spinal tap, also known as a lumbar puncture, is a procedure in which a long needle is inserted into the spinal canal in the lower back to withdraw cerebrospinal fluid. The fluid can be tested for infection and signs of inflammation. In my case, it would be examined for certain proteins seen in most patients with MS.

"Well, I think it'd be preferable to have a definite diagnosis before we start medication," Dr. Reynard replied.

Okay. I agreed. We needed to be sure. A spinal tap would be next.

CHAPTER 9:

A Life Sentence

November 2009

The needle for a lumbar puncture is almost as long as a pencil used to keep score in a game of minigolf. Hollow, with a beveled tip, it's the sort of needle a proud cartoon doctor would wave in front of an uncooperative child, threatening him to "settle down, or else. . . ." As a resident, I learned to do spinal taps on patients in the ER or admitted to the hospital suspected of having a neurologic condition, like meningitis, but I was never very proficient and hadn't even watched the procedure since finishing my medical training.

My lumbar puncture was to be done under fluoroscopy, using an x-ray beam to provide the radiologist with a real-time picture of my spine to guide the needle to the right place. I noted the needle on the tray of instruments next to the table, before I settled into position on the white sheet, and tried to erase the image.

"This won't take long," the radiologist said.

"I just want to get it over with," I said.

I thought of the teenager we tapped during my residency at the University of Cincinnati. She had come to the ER with headaches. We diagnosed her with pseudotumor cerebri, also known as idiopathic intracranial hypertension—a condition caused by increased pressure from a buildup of spinal fluid inside the skull. Was she scared? Did anyone explain to her what was happening? If only I could go back, I would be more patient, more reassuring, and a lot more informative.

The test itself was no worse than getting a mole removed. After the injection with lidocaine, I could feel only a mild pressure when the giant needle entered my back. In just a few minutes, we were done.

"That's it?" I asked when the radiologist pushed back on his stool, holding two or three small tubes filled with clear liquid.

"Nothing to it," he said. "Usually it takes a week or so to get the results back. You know, we're looking for oligoclonal bands, the proteins that help diagnose MS. It takes a while."

"Okay. I figured."

"You may have a headache. If it's bad, it could indicate a spinal fluid leak, which we can fix with a blood patch. I know it sounds weird, but it usually works pretty well."

He explained that, if needed, a small amount of blood could be injected in the space around the spinal canal. After about thirty minutes, it would clot and seal off the leak. Although I'm told such precautions are no longer necessary, he also instructed me to lie flat for the next twenty-four hours to reduce the chance of a headache.

I was the ideal patient, following the doctor's orders perfectly. My sister, Cathy, always ready to jump in with whatever I needed, came to help with the kids, who adored her. Another friend brought veggie lasagna from Pasta and Company for dinner. My parents called from Washington, DC, where they lived and worked during the week, to check on me. Don cleaned up after dinner and put both kids to bed. We thought the worst was over.

The next morning I awoke, relieved to find that, despite continued dizziness, I was headache-free. Soon I'd be back on my feet, chasing kids and examining patients. I made my way downstairs. Since I couldn't exercise, I decided just to stay in my pajamas and pretend all this lounging around was my choice. I stretched out on the couch again, tucked myself in with a fluffy blanket, and picked up the remote, flipping through morning news programs before settling on HGTV.

Don brought me granola and yogurt for breakfast. "How do you feel?" he asked.

"Okay," I said. "I'm going to just stay camped out here all day, and hopefully by this evening, I can do whatever I want."

I spent the day flipping through channels on the TV, sorting mail, and becoming reacquainted with boredom, after a long separation. Boredom and I were not good friends. Even as a kid, I always found something to do. I would rediscover a forgotten toy, read a book, organize my desk. I remembered one day visiting family in El Paso over winter break. Cathy, my cousins, and I tired of our games, and the weather kept us inside. We watched five movies in one day. I didn't want to watch five movies again.

I turned on my laptop to deal with e-mails from work, challenging myself to reduce my inbox to thirty, then twenty e-mails. I tried to distract myself from thoughts of MS and its implications, from my growing conviction that my dizziness was never going away. But instead of improving as the day progressed, I got worse. That evening, I felt exhausted and couldn't eat dinner. I thought maybe lying on the coach all day was contributing to my malaise. I would feel better once I was back on my feet.

On the second day after the spinal tap, I went for a short jog in the neighborhood. *Mind over matter,* I told myself, tying my tennis shoes and heading out the door. *I am going to ignore feeling bad, and maybe I will stop feeling bad.*

It didn't work. As I approached our house at the end of my usual route, I felt like I was running in a swimming pool, struggling with each slow movement. Usually running helped my mood and energy. Not this time.

On day three, post–spinal tap, I didn't try to run. It was Sunday, and Don had to work again. "You'll be okay?" he asked, grabbing his white doctor coat off a hook by the door.

"I'm done being sick," I replied. "I'll be fine. I'm taking the kids to breakfast with my mom and Cathy. And Beth is here from Dallas. Then we're going Christmas shopping."

"Sounds good. Don't overdo it, though, okay?" Don gave me a quick hug and headed to his car.

Buoyed by thoughts of a Mexican breakfast at Curra's restaurant with my family, I tried to ignore my dizziness and mild nausea as I got the kids dressed to go out. But by the time we arrived at the restaurant, my façade of health had started to fade. After a round of hugs, I sat down across from Cathy and my cousin Beth, with Clara on one side of me and Ella on the other. My mom sat at the end of the table next to Clara.

Beth's visits were always a treat. Just ten months younger than me, she was full of positive energy and funny stories. When she came to town, we would celebrate, even without a birthday or holiday, picking up veggie burgers from Phil's Icehouse and an assortment from Hey Cupcake for a picnic on my back patio. She would bring little gifts: candles, lavender hand cream, homemade cookies. She, Cathy, and I would take long walks in Pease Park and catch up on family gossip.

Now Beth looked at me with concern, her brow furrowed.

"You're not feeling good. I can tell," she said as a waitress handed us menus and poured a round of ice water.

"I'm trying, but it's not going particularly well," I said.

"That's really hard," Cathy said. "It was already hard trying to balance your work and the kids. . . ." My younger sister always understood. I appreciated her sympathy and validation.

"It just takes time," my mom chimed in. "You'll get better."

My mom, ever the optimist, wasn't quite convinced I had MS. She held out hope that the spinal tap might turn out to be normal, my diagnosis a false alarm. My mom combined her positive nature with an astonishing work ethic and stamina. A nationally known advocate for children, she was tireless in leading the charge for universal prekindergarten across the country. To those around her, she was a stalwart who didn't take no for an answer. To me, she was Superwoman and my best friend. I wanted to believe her, to be persuaded that I was healthy and strong and resilient. I wanted to. But I didn't.

"I don't want this," Clara said, pushing away her water.

"You don't have to have water, Clara. I'm going to order you some fruit and a tortilla. You'll like that," I told her. I handed her some paper and crayons. "Can you draw me a picture?"

I looked at the menu—breakfast tacos, *migas, huevos rancheros.* Clara scribbled on the paper, and Ella played with some Wikki Stix my sister had brought for her.

"Are you okay?" my mom asked. "Is there anything that looks good?"

No. Nothing looks good. Curra's was an Austin institution. I loved it, but that day I couldn't eat. I looked up at my mom. "I don't want anything right now."

Clara begged for more paper, but I didn't have any. I gave her a napkin. The noise of the crowded restaurant, the smell of Mexican food, and Clara's whining were too much. I put my head on the table. *Who am I kidding? I'm not better,* I thought. I felt worse than ever. My positive attitude wasn't helping. Optimism was a burden, leading to disappointment and an innate pressure to be okay when I wasn't. I couldn't go Christmas shopping. I couldn't do anything.

"I need to lie down," I said. "I thought I'd be okay, but I'm feeling sick again."

Serenaded by a chorus of "I'm sorrys" from my family, I left the table to go to the car. There I sat on the passenger side, my head resting against the window. *This sucks. This wasn't supposed to happen.*

My mom came out with the kids a few minutes later and insisted on driving me home.

"I wanted to spend the day with you all," I said, barely able to raise my voice above a whisper.

"You're going to feel better, and there will be other opportunities to spend time together," my mom said. She strapped both kids into their car seats. I continued to lean against the passenger door, longing to be home.

Five minutes after leaving the restaurant, as we rounded a corner near the Long Center, across from the lake, I suddenly sat up straight. "I'm going to be sick."

My mom pulled over. I shoved open the car door and dashed to the gutter, vomiting into damp leaves and trash before collapsing on the ground. My chest felt heavy and tight, and my throat burned. I rolled to one side, wishing I could sink into the soggy grass, surrendering completely. Meanwhile, Ella and Clara jostled in their car seats, impatient, oblivious. My mom rolled down her window, calling from the driver's seat to see if I was okay. I wasn't.

In a soupy fog of dizziness, I caught a glimpse across the street at the lake. Three weeks before, I had been jogging around that lake, Lady Bird Lake, the gravel crunching under my Brooks running shoes. I had pushed a double jogging stroller, loaded with my two kids, who laughed and snacked on raisins and animal crackers, counting the dogs as we passed. I had surveyed the skyline as we neared downtown, noting the cranes, the progress on a new office building by the South First Street bridge and another near Lamar Boulevard. The lake was my haven, my favorite part of the city. Now, as I struggled to stand and stagger back to the car, the lake seemed to taunt me: Look at you now. Aren't you glad you spent so much time running? A lot of good that did you!

"Lisa, are you okay? I'm really concerned about you," my mom repeated as I fell back into the car.

"I don't know," I mumbled. "I think I just need to get home."

We dropped off the kids with a sitter near my house, and then my mom drove me home. She helped me—weak, trembling—climb the stairs to my bedroom, and she brought me a glass of water.

"Is there anything else I can do?" she asked. "I feel bad leaving you like this."

"No. Just go and enjoy your time with Cathy and Beth."

"I'll pick up the kids from the babysitter's at 1 o'clock. I can keep them as long as you need me to after that," she said.

I burrowed under the covers as waves of more dizziness and nausea rushed over me. My head felt thick and full, like a saturated sponge. I was enormously relieved to be in bed but devastated to miss this rare weekend with my mom, sister, and much-loved cousin.

My bedroom was cool, but the humidity from the steady drizzle outside created a clamminess that made the sheets moist and uncomfortable. I felt tears in my eyes—a welling up of self-pity—and again wondered how I had come to this moment. I wasn't supposed to get sick.

Don called from the hospital to check on me.

"How many times have you thrown up? Do you have a headache?" he asked, launching into doctor mode. "A headache could indicate a spinal leak and explain why you're feeling bad. You'd need a blood patch."

"I have a slight headache, probably from puking. But I don't think this is a spinal leak," I muttered.

"Do you need to go to the ER for IV fluids?" he asked.

"No, I just need to rest, I guess."

A dark depression hung over me for two days. On Monday I tried to go for a walk but had to climb back in bed. I tried to go to work but had to come home to rest. During my more optimistic moments, I thought my depression might be a heavy curtain just about to lift, but most of the time, it seemed like an impenetrable wall. I was facing a life sentence with MS. It was inescapable. How could I ever feel normal again?

I didn't want to reveal the depth of my depression to Don. I knew it would just make him irritable and discouraged. He was struggling to care for the kids on his own, to anticipate and address their needs without me as backup. He periodically came to check on me, sad and worried, though trying to put on a brave face.

On Monday night Don pulled out an inspirational book to read together—*Kitchen Table Wisdom*. The book's author, Rachel Naomi Remen, is a wise physician and author who writes of her personal health difficulties with Crohn's disease as well as her encounters with hospice patients. Her stories of other people struggling and ultimately making peace with adversity hinted that my life wasn't over, that I might be stronger than I thought. "In my experience, life can change abruptly and end without warning, but life is not fragile," Remen wrote.

Fragile. That was what I was feeling. It was a new F-word for me, and I didn't like it. Not one bit. We read on, about tenacity, which she thought existed at the intracellular level. I liked the idea of it, but whether I could ever harness that innate tenacity . . . well, let's just say I had my doubts.

Don gave me a pep talk. "I know you had a horrible weekend, but you're still recovering from the spinal tap," he said. "I think it's pretty likely you'll feel better . . . like soon."

"I thought I was supposed to feel better the next day. Maybe it's not the tap, but this is what it feels like to have MS," I said.

"When you're sick, it always seems like you'll never get better. That's the worst. But you will. You'll get better."

Don reminded me what Dr. Reynard had told us: With treatment, I had an 80 percent chance of doing well ten years postdiagnosis with no to minimal symptoms. Thanks to years of research producing new miracle drugs, I would not end up like Mr. Sloane.

"We'll get through this together," he said. "I'm betting tomorrow you'll feel a little better."

He was right. The next morning, my dizziness had receded. I wasn't back to normal, but I felt like I had found the stairs to exit the dungeon. Don and I celebrated that glimmer of hope, with rare smiles, hesitant jokes. We even dared to discuss the upcoming holidays. By the end of the week, when I gathered with my family to celebrate Thanksgiving, I felt genuinely better and tremendously grateful.

And when Dr. Reynard called with the spinal tap results a few nights later, confirming my MS diagnosis, I listened to my instructions to start the new medication he was prescribing. Then I walked into the kitchen to tell Don and share a hug with him. We were expecting these results. We knew what was wrong. At last, we had regained some sense of control. We had a plan, and I had a smart doctor and medicine on the way. We could cope. After summoning the kids to the dinner table, Don turned on the stereo, and we listened to Bob Marley sing, reminding us that everything would be alright.

CHAPTER 10

The Most Wonderful Time of the Year

December 2009

Not only was I *that* mom—the one to obsess over packing school snacks and lunches, to sign my kids up for toddler gymnastics and music lessons, and to insist on perfect orange icing for Clara's birthday cake—apparently, we were *that* family. The one that sends the too-long holiday letter, complete with photos of smiling children. Don and I would tag-team our efforts: I would write the year-in-review, and he would make it funny. "We took a trip to San Francisco for a medical conference," I had written in our last missive. "Unfortunately," Don added, "Ella didn't sleep well, or perhaps was temporarily possessed by demons. Either way, it gave us a better understanding of the need for child abandonment laws."

I didn't want to write the letter that year. I was grieving for Christmas past, for every little thing I had taken for granted. *Was it only a couple of months back that we had made plans for Don's parents to visit? And I had started buying stocking stuffers, priding myself on getting an early start?* That seemed a lifetime away. All I had to look forward to now were MRIs, co-pays, and God knows what type of new and frightening symptoms. I was a planner. A doer. A take-the-bull-by-the-horns kind of person (a Texas metaphor if ever there was one). Now there was only uncertainty. And dread.

Don and I imagined future letters describing a search for caregivers, goodbyes to jobs, to travel, to favorite things. Maybe we'd downplay those fears with an uncomfortable joke about disabled parking. But what about this year? Our family and friends expected to hear from us. Not writing the letter would indicate a shift, an admission that more had changed than we wanted to believe. We faced up to it as best we could.

"It hasn't been the easiest year," we wrote. "The most difficult news, as you may know, is that Lisa was diagnosed with multiple sclerosis in November. Obviously, this is something neither of us wished to welcome into our lives." That out of the way, we boasted about Ella's stellar gift-wrapping skills and shared a story of Clara beheading her doll.

More than anything, our update was a thank-you to those who had helped us—to the friends who sent cards and e-mails, brought dinner, arranged playdates for the kids. Our support circle had rallied, and we wanted to show our appreciation.

But first I needed stamps.

"Here we are!" I said to the kids as we pulled into the post office parking lot, feigning enthusiasm for a chore I mostly dreaded. I *mostly* dreaded it because I knew that the lines would be horrible, and I would be impatient, and taking the kids anywhere was invariably difficult. But this errand also brought a little spark of holiday nostalgia. It was a connection to the past, a glimmer of hope.

The line for the automated machine was much shorter than the line leading up to an actual human postal worker, but it was still daunting. I took my place at the end, shifting Clara to my left side and letting go of her sister's hand. Ella stayed next to me until she caught sight of the Santa decorations on a window near the door and wandered toward them. Clara was squirming. "Down!" she commanded. I set her on the scuffed tile floor, holding her hand as best I could.

I watched as the person first in line pulled package after package out of her big plastic bag. It reminded me of a magic trick I'd seen at Esther's Follies, a popular sketch comedy club in downtown Austin. In the act, just when you thought the bag was empty, one more impossibly large item was removed—an umbrella, a crutch, a set of golf clubs. But this woman didn't have a magician's finesse and speed. She kept pushing buttons on the automated machine, sighing in exasperation, inserting her credit card—after several minutes of fussing over the machine—slapping a sticker on the package, and pulling out another box. I was sure the golf clubs must be in there somewhere.

The girls were antsy. Having freed herself from my grasp, Clara joined her sister near the decorations, pointing, shouting, "Santa!" Ella tried to pick her up, but Clara resisted, and they barely missed being smashed by the automatic door.

"Clara, sweetie, come here!" I said, noting that now two more people had gathered behind me in line.

Clara ignored me. She ran across the room, unconstrained, laughing. She narrowly avoided a collision with the woman who had finally finished with her packages, the one I now thought of as "Esther." Clara slowed for a second, reaching down to peel a sticky white thing off the dirty floor, a stray packing label most likely. I reminded myself to wipe Clara's hands as soon as we got back to the car.

"Frosty the Snowman" blared through unseen speakers, and I tried to decipher all the words so I could sing it, at Ella's request, later that evening. Remembering the old cartoon movie from childhood, I pictured Frosty, racing through the snowy village, chased by joyful children. This was no village, but it hadn't stopped Clara from turning into Frosty, dashing around the post office, getting increasingly giddy in parallel with my own escalating embarrassment. After nearly slipping on the floor, she jumped behind a pair of orange cones connected by plastic netting that blocked a dark section of the post office under renovation.

She was oblivious, disobedient, wild. I was inattentive, incompetent. Surely that's what everyone was thinking.

"Clara, you're not supposed to go back there," I said in a voice I hoped was firm but still cheerful.

She skipped out from behind the barricade, then jumped back in again, taunting me. I grabbed Ella's hand. "Help me catch your sister," I whispered. Then I turned to the person behind me, mumbling, "One sec."

I stepped away, mortified, to scoop up my unruly child.

"Clara! This isn't a game!" I lunged, grabbing her around the waist and carrying her sideways, screaming, back to the line.

As my upside-down child struggled to escape, I stepped back out of the line into view of the people in front of me. Everyone had things to do, and I didn't like to ask for favors. I was ashamed. But I was dizzy, worn-out, desperate. "I'm so sorry, but could I possibly go next?" I asked, hoisting Clara up again. "I'm just getting stamps. No packages. It'll just take a second." I smiled—grimaced, really—hoping that I didn't come across as needy or, worse, entitled.

The young woman at the front of the line pulled a fancy wallet from her fancy handbag and fiddled with some bills. Looking at me, she shrugged. "That's all I'm getting too," she said, then turned her back on me.

Of course. This is the way my life is now, the way it will always be.

I was near tears.

Have mercy, I silently pleaded. *I can't control these kids, but I'm trying. I have MS. Each day I wake up terrified.* I wanted to ask her to show a little charity, to remind her that it was Christmas, that maybe one day she might need help, and the laws of karma were not on her side.

I also wanted to punch her in the face.

As a child I was devastated to learn that Santa Claus isn't real. As an adult I discovered long ago that the perfect Christmas isn't real either. It can never live up to the hype and expectation. This year, the constant reminder of how the holidays were supposed to be was especially irritating and disheartening. It made reality seem inadequate, highlighting my deficiencies, scolding me if I didn't live in a state of constant merriment.

Don and I had supported each other during those first few weeks after my MS diagnosis, strengthening our marriage and bringing us closer. He made dinner and came with me to doctors' appointments. His pep talks had helped me gain perspective. But stress was a constant presence threatening to unravel us. By mid-December, he stopped sending his midday check-in texts. As usual during the winter months, his work at the hospital had increased, with the return of flu, respiratory syncytial virus (RSV), and other cold-season infections. Kids were getting sick, and Don and his colleagues were swamped. There was no *ping* to remind me to "Hang in there" or to ask how my day was going. I couldn't blame him. We were exhausted with no reserves left.

My in-laws could hardly have picked a worse time to arrive. As I tried to straighten up in preparation for their visit, I feared our house-keeping had reached a new low. Piles of junk had materialized in every corner: socks, coins, Legos, game pieces, paper, blocks. There must have been, literally, one million things.

"Really, Lisa?" Don had asked. "*Literally* one million things?"

"Yes," I snapped. "I counted them. One million even."

As I shopped for Christmas gifts, I wondered: *Is it really a selling point when a toy advertises "Over two hundred pieces!" Like that's supposed to make me want it?* "Only six pieces that all stick together or evaporate when left out of their box" would be a far more attractive feature.

Don's parents, with the best of intentions, came loaded down with gifts—at least eight perfect packages for each child. This, despite our earlier conversation about "cutting back," despite my trotting out that really lame line, "The nicest gift of all is having you join us for Christmas."

I am not going to say anything, I told myself. *They are warm and generous. They are wonderful with the kids. Don's mom will wash dishes, chop vegetables, and fold laundry without being asked. I am going to be grateful.*

For Christmas Eve we had planned to drive out to Lake Travis, but a cold front blew in that morning with howling winds, littering the yard with branches and leaves. *The yard, which had just been cleaned, now looked like our house with the million things,* I thought as I soothed fussy Clara—who was sick with a cold—and helped Ella find her blue winter jacket. Realizing that our trip to the lake would be about as pleasant as a picnic in a meat locker, Don announced that instead he would take everyone to the new Disney movie, *The Princess and the Frog*, at the mall.

"Don, Clara is sick!" I'd said. "I can't take her to a movie. And she's too little anyway."

"Well, can your mom keep her?"

"No, I don't think that's fair to ask," I said. "Clara's super clingy, and my mom is busy getting ready to host us tonight. I'll just have to skip the movie and stay home with Clara."

"Well, what do you want me to do?" Don asked. He had been on edge all morning. His parents' arrival had amped up his anxiety. He still worried that his father and I would get into a fight about politics. He was also triggered by his mother's conviction that Clara was on the verge of a fatal accident every time she climbed on the furniture.

"You can't do anything else. Just go to the movie. Hopefully, Clara will take a nap, and I can finish some last-minute gift wrapping," I said.

Soon after Don departed with his parents and Ella, the music and lights all snapped off at once. Clara looked up in surprise.

"Well, this is just what I was hoping for!" I said.

Apparently, the wind was to blame for the power outage. Gusts of forty miles per hour accompanied the cold front, dropping temperatures over twenty degrees. The house was getting chilly. I didn't want to build a fire because I didn't trust Clara to keep her distance, and I wanted to avoid a safety lecture when Don and his parents returned. I pulled out an extra sweater to stay warm and put a little fleece jacket on Clara. Then I created a new pile of junk in the kitchen when I cleaned off our breakfast table to make room for Play-Doh.

I opened a brand-new container of orange Play-Doh and handed Clara a rolling pin. She pulled out the orange Play-Doh and promptly mixed it with the old green Play-Doh, as she shaped "cookies." I started sorting through one of the many junk piles, but after three or four minutes, Clara slipped out of her chair and, in a whiny voice, asked to be lifted up. She was already done with her cookies.

The house got colder. The fierce wind reminded me more of Austin's spring thunderstorms than the holidays. I half expected lightning and pouring rain.

After two long hours the power finally came back on. "Hooray!" I shouted. "Come on, Clara. Let's turn on the Christmas tree lights!" Clara followed me into the living room and reached for the cord.

"No, baby, I need to do that," I said, snatching the cord from her.

"I want to!" Clara whined, trying to get the cord away from me.

"I know, but it's not safe." I plugged in the lights, lifted my now-crying child, and headed back to the kitchen where I gave her some applesauce. Then I turned on the Christmas radio station. After a slew of annoying commercials, I heard the first few notes of the song that epitomizes holiday cheer: "It's the Most Wonderful Time of the Year."

"Ugh!" I said to Clara. "This again. This is the reason I see so many people with anxiety and depression over the holidays." I remembered them well: the stressed mom who couldn't afford presents for her young son; the families separated by distance or even death; the middle-aged woman with high blood pressure who confided her suicidal thoughts to me, tearing up because she couldn't visit her adult daughter in Minnesota. Thinking of her, I tried to appreciate my situation. My Christmas would be full of family—noisy, crowded. My patient yearned to see her daughter and couldn't. Yet here I was with my own daughter, wishing for some alone time. I reminded myself that Don would be home soon.

"More!" Clara said, pointing at her empty bowl of applesauce.

Andy Williams carried on about glowing hearts, loved ones, and mistletoe. It was too much, and I pushed the off button.

"This song sets up this ridiculous expectation, like there's something wrong with us if we're not super happy," I said to my two-year-old as I scooped more applesauce into her bowl. "If this is the most wonderful time of the year, I just want to go crawl into a cave."

Don arrived home after more than four hours.

"Where have you been? I've been trying to call you," I said. Clara had *not* napped. I had *not* had time to wrap gifts.

"I know. We were in the movie, and I couldn't answer my phone," Don replied. He looked exhausted—like he'd just worked a thirty-six-hour shift at the hospital.

"And the movie was four hours long?" I asked.

"No," he said, sighing with irritation. "According to the *Austin Chronicle*, the movie started at 11:10, but when we arrived at the theater, we found out it was actually at 12:45."

"And you couldn't call me to explain that?"

"I didn't think of it. We had to get lunch, and we had to get Ella some mittens. . . ."

"What? Why? She already has mittens!"

"Well, I didn't know that. She couldn't find any mittens today when we were leaving. . . . It's just mittens," he said.

One million and two things.

The wind had dissipated by the time we loaded the kids in their matching red dresses and my in-laws into the car for the drive to my parents' house for Christmas Eve dinner. My mom welcomed us at the kitchen door, setting down a pot of mashed potatoes and hugging all of us. My dad followed suit, cheerful, greeting everyone with enthusiasm. I wanted to celebrate this special night, but disappointments, small and large, competed for my attention: *Clara's still sick, I forgot to wear my Christmas earrings, I have MS.* I tried to enjoy the festive house, full of excited children and favorite foods. I tried to pretend it was Christmas as usual. *Who am I kidding?*

Back at home, I put the kids to bed alone, going through the usual routine of teeth brushing and bedtime stories.

"Santa can't come until y'all are asleep," I told the girls, and Ella nodded solemnly. She went to bed without a fuss. When I finally escaped from Clara's room, hoping she would sleep, I was dismayed to find Don lying on our bed in the dark. Light seeped in from the hallway, but it was still too dark for me to see his expression. I closed the door and turned on the light.

"What's going on?" I asked. "Are you going to sleep?"

"I was going to try," he said, shielding his eyes from the light. "Can you turn that off?"

"Turn it off? No. We've got work to do," I said. "Weren't you going to help me?"

"With what?" he asked, groggy, annoyed.

"Are you kidding me?" I said, my voice rising. "It's Christmas Eve!"

"So? I'm exhausted," he said. "What else do you want from me?"

I realized he was genuinely confused. "Oh my God. Seriously? All the Santa stuff? What the hell! I'll just do all that by myself, too."

I didn't wait for his response. I stumbled down the stairs in tears, grabbed my car keys, and left. I didn't have a jacket, but I didn't care. I just needed to get out of that miserable house.

"Have a Holly, Jolly Christmas!" belted out from the radio when

I turned on the car. "Oh my God!" I moaned, switching the radio off and backing out of the driveway into the dark street. The bright Christmas lights in our front yard brought fresh tears to my eyes. *This is supposed to be the highlight of the year!* It's supposed to be fun to fill children's stockings. The girls were getting new bicycles. I had envisioned Don bringing them in from the garage and us setting them up in front of the tree together, admiring the idyllic scene. Instead, I was driving down cold, deserted streets, wondering if our marriage could survive Christmas, let alone my MS.

We had struggled even before my diagnosis. As I drove, I remembered our disagreement about the movie from earlier in the day—the mix-up over the time and Don's failure to call. I catalogued the fights of the previous year, too many to count—a blowup while prepping for a picnic, a shouting match when Don forgot to share a schedule change, so many squabbles over bedtime routines, grumpy moods, and who emptied the dishwasher more.

I thought of the ruined summer evening in the backyard when Don yelled at me in response to my question about our shared cell-phone charger. "It's upstairs, and I want it to stay upstairs!" We then performed our usual little skit: "Change your tone." "No, you change *your* tone." "No, I said it first. You change *your* tone!"

The repetitive nature of this fight, its predictability and inevitability, made it all the more infuriating. Clara had interrupted by proudly presenting me with a smooshed caterpillar she had scooped off the parsley plant in our herb garden. When I saw it, I burst into tears, turning away from her startled face. Ella and I had spotted the little yellow and black caterpillar the previous week. Every day we had been checking on it to see how much it had grown. Now it was a glob of slime in Clara's hand.

It's symbolic of our marriage, I had thought at the time. And as

I drove away from our house on Christmas Eve, I felt certain I had been right. We thought we were building something beautiful, but we couldn't partner around child-rearing or even share a cell phone charger.

We can't even help each other play Santa Claus.

I pulled up in front of my parents' house, calling from the car to give them a heads-up. My mom greeted me in her bathrobe and gave me a hug. I wanted to cling to her but didn't want to appear too fragile, too needy. She was resilient—less bothered by the disappointments and imperfections that weighed me down. Still, I didn't want to spoil her vision of how Christmas was supposed to be.

My mom led me into the kitchen. The house was dark, with just one light on above the sink, but, in sharp contrast to my sink, it was clean and orderly. I couldn't believe we'd just had a party there.

"I'm so sorry," I said, still crying. "I hated to bother you, but I just had to get away."

"It's been a hard couple of months for you all," she said. "What can I do? Can I make you some tea?"

"Yeah, that'd be great," I said.

I sat down at the table near the kitchen and took a deep breath. "I can't believe Don wasn't going to help me put out the Santa stuff."

"He's just worn-out, Lisa. It's hard for him to have you getting sick. His job is hard, too. . . . Now you're hosting his parents."

She turned on the electric kettle and handed me a sampling of different tea options. I selected ginger peach.

"It's hard for you, too," she continued. "Having guests and not feeling good."

I drank the tea and sat there with my mom, glad to be in that calm, quiet place. She was right, as usual. Don and I were maxed out. We were still processing my diagnosis, and we could barely handle our kids. Don was racing back and forth between the hospital and our house, now trying to ensure his parents were comfortable, and feeling exhausted all the time.

"You've got those two precious girls," she said, smiling. "They looked adorable in their Christmas dresses tonight. That Clara—she's something else."

"I know, thanks," I said, not ready to smile yet. "I'm sorry she made a mess in the playroom. I think I forgot to clean it up."

"Oh, that's okay. She's just being a two-year-old," she said.

We sat there together. I enjoyed the silence, interspersed by my mom's musings about the kids and plans for brunch the next day.

"I think I need to go back," I finally said, taking a last sip of tea. I was fortified now. I could face Don, the million things, and my children again.

"Is there anything else I can do?"

"No, this is really what I needed," I said, giving her a hug again and picking up my keys from the kitchen counter.

Don was waiting for me at home. I found him downstairs in the kitchen, replacing a trash bag. "I forgot about the Christmas stuff. I can help now," he said.

I still held on to some lingering strands of anger, but I knew I had to let go. As much as I felt sorry for myself, I was beginning to feel sorry for him, too. He was stressed, drained, demoralized. I could definitely relate. And it was Christmas Eve—not a night for fights. I let out a deep breath. "Okay, thanks," I said. "The kids are definitely asleep, right?"

"Yeah, I just checked again."

"Okay, good. Can you bring in the bikes?" I asked.

"Sure," he said, turning to get his shoes and head out to the garage.

I went upstairs to pull down the boxes of stocking stuffers from the top of our armoire. The joy was gone for me, but at least we could fake it for the kids. I carried the boxes downstairs and took down Clara's red and green stocking, carefully filling it with little metal cars, Band-Aids, and ponytail holders, with a Curious George monkey peeking out of the top. I loaded Ella's with watercolor paints, markers, and bubble bath, topped off with a spotted-cow stuffed animal and two colorful candy canes. Don brought in the small bikes—both a shiny purple—and seeing them again did make me smile a little.

"If we can get our act together, I think the kids are gonna have a good Christmas," I said.

And they did, for the most part. The bikes and stocking stuffers were a hit. Don complained about the amount of stuff we amassed from friends and family members. Ella's demands for more, more, *more* presents drove me mad, though I reassured myself her behavior was age appropriate and not another parental failure. Don's mother was distressed with Clara's clear preference for her grandpa; Clara wasn't subtle or polite, repeating, "No like Grandma." But we kept the shouting and crying to a reasonable level.

I crawled into bed that night, feeling relieved. And as I drifted off to sleep, I rewrote the lyrics to those Christmas songs that had been driving me crazy. Nothing captured my mishmash of feelings: disillusionment with still a little bit of hope and gratitude. It didn't have the right ring to it, but I settled on "It's the most joy/stressful time of the year."

CHAPTER 11:

Sex, Drugs, and How 'bout Staying in School?

January 2010

R eturning to work after the holidays was a welcome distraction. It forced me to tamp down my fears and help my patients, many of whom were struggling with challenges beyond my comprehension: a son arrested for selling drugs, a hand mangled from a band-saw accident, severe vision loss after another work accident. Was it wrong to compare myself to others, to note that I was fortunate, even with my recent diagnosis?

I never sought out tales of woe to make myself feel better, but my patients' stories did put my own issues in perspective—perhaps too much so. Because their needs eclipsed mine, I considered my own pain trivial, fueling my inner drill sergeant—the same force that compelled me to exercise even when I felt unwell, to respond to every e-mail I received, and to go to work even when my dizziness made me want to flop on the couch. Now, in typical fashion, I told myself to stop this self-absorbed wallowing and get over it. I never would have judged a patient or a friend with such harshness. I would have recognized her fear for what it was. But I wasn't the most compassionate person when it came to myself. Staying busy was the best coping technique I could muster.

Although my self-pity dissipated, and even my dizziness continued to evaporate, my overwhelming task list led to loud complaining. "I'm getting a hundred e-mails a day, and somehow I'm still supposed to see patients, and I'm still catching up from Christmas, and even from being off work back in November," I lamented to Don, arriving home later than I'd promised and collapsing into a kitchen chair. He was nice enough to ignore the fact that I had forgotten to say hello or hug the kids.

"Half of my patients no-showed today, but I'm still late because I had to work someone in at the end of the day, and she took forever, and she wouldn't go to the ER for this horrible abdominal pain. I didn't know if her pain was really, like, a serious thing or if she was totally blowing it out of proportion. I feel bad even for saying that, but sometimes it's so hard to know."

Don, who had recovered from his holiday depression, was tossing our dinner salad, but he signaled with a slight movement of his free hand that I needed to snap out of it. It was subtle, but I understood. Only then did I notice Ella, who was trying to show me an intricate three-dimensional collage she had made at school.

Part of my problem was lack of sleep. Both kids had been getting us up so often that I was used to awakening at 2:00 AM, wondering which child would come in next. Even when the kids slept all night, I suffered from terrible insomnia, feeding my anxiety and bad attitude.

Don gave me a little speech a couple of days later. "Lisa, okay, like I know this really sucks. I get that you can't sleep and that the not sleeping makes everything extra hard. But you're being so negative all the time. It makes everything so much harder. It doesn't help our family, and in the end, you know, it doesn't help you either."

I sighed, rolling my eyes. "What am I supposed to do? You seem to think I can just turn on some sort of positivity switch."

I wanted him to validate my frustration, to sit with me in that swamp of negativity for a bit. Why couldn't he just tell me it was okay to be angry? Why couldn't he be angry, too? I know he was trying to guide me. I know he was trying to help. He knew me well, and his sympathy was real and deep. But he had that guy thing that wanted desperately to fix everything, to regain control. He was seeking the formula for normalcy. He was going for calm and content. But I felt criticized.

"I wish you hadn't gotten MS." He paused as if to acknowledge how obvious his statement was. "You know I'd do anything to make it go away. I mean, do I have to even say that?"

"That would be nice," I said.

"I just think you should try not to be so negative around the kids. And what about your patients? I imagine this happens at work, too," he said.

Don was on my side. I knew that, but I still wanted to lash out.

"What do you want me to say?" I asked, not even trying to hide my frustration.

"Just think about it. You have to ask if it's making things better," he added.

Don sounded more like an HR manager than a husband. But a part of me—the part not clenched in resentment and why me's—knew he was right. I needed to figure out how to turn my self-pity into compassion—for my patients and myself.

I had been unprofessional that day, grumbling to Terri when I saw that Ruth Simms was on my schedule again. She would be complaining of back pain, still smoking two packs a day, and grumbling about everything and everyone. Talk about negativity! "What's the point?" I'd snapped. "She never does anything I recommend."

"Can I see her for you?" Terri had offered, cheerful and supportive as always.

"No, it's okay. Just have two units of packed red blood cells to transfuse me when I'm done with her. She's a total vampire patient and will suck me dry."

But how do you just snap out of it when *it* is a chronic disease? I told myself again that MS was no big deal, that I should count my blessings and get over it. But that approach—no matter how stoic—denied the reality of the sadness we faced. MS was a burden, and I was entitled to be angry. I had spent my life doing everything I could to stay healthy, doing what I had been told were all the right things. I hadn't counted on something as simple and unpredictable as bad luck.

We try, in medicine, to make predictions. Calculating a Framingham heart risk score, I can tell someone their odds of heart disease. With the Gail Model, I can estimate the chance of breast cancer. We analyze DNA, looking for clues to someone's fate. My risk for chronic disease was low by all measures. Even our best tools are badly flawed. We seek explanations, but most of the time, disease strikes at random. Eventually, our bodies will betray us. We know this, but still we are surprised by illness. Much of the time, we don't see it coming.

Still, I wasn't entitled to take it out on other people. I needed to find a way to honor my disappointment but then to shut it down, wall it off, let it go. I couldn't let MS define who I was.

Easier said than done.

⌒

Don's advice came back to me the next day at the clinic as Sara Maria handed me the intake forms for my next two patients, a brother and sister, who were there for well-child checks. I had kind of hoped they would no-show so that I'd have time to catch up on e-mail and other administrative tasks—the type of work that doesn't seem important until it goes undone. But channeling Don, I nodded to Sara Maria, took the forms, and replied, "Great, thank you." I put on my white coat, grabbed an extra pen, and headed into the exam room.

Diego was a cute little boy, just a few months older than Ella. His Cookie Monster T-shirt was a little faded and his jeans were too big, requiring him to hitch them up periodically. He returned my smile, which grew broader when I handed him a book—a story called *Wolf!* It had been donated by Reach Out and Read, a national nonprofit that encourages parents to read with their children daily—an important activity that promotes literacy, language acquisition, and brain development. I had applied for us to become a partner clinic the year before. Now, giving out books during well-child exams was a favorite part of my job.

"This book is for you to take home and keep," I said in Spanish. "Do you like to read?"

Diego nodded.

"Me too. I hope you'll read every day with your mom, or maybe your sister."

Diego was there with his mother—a woman in her mid-thirties, wearing a light blue uniform, probably for a hotel cleaning company or laundromat. His teenage sister, Esperanza, sat slumped in the chair, picking at her fingernails. Glancing at her, I thought, *Yeah, she's not going to read to her little brother.* Oh well. I would have to deal with her next, but for now, my focus was on Diego.

After reviewing some basic medical history with his mom, I turned back to Diego. "Do you like Cookie Monster?" I asked.

He nodded with a shy smile.

"I do, too. And Big Bird," I said. I stretched out my stethoscope for his inspection. "Do you know what this is for?"

He nodded again. "For my heart."

"You're right! I'm going to listen to your heart, and then, if you want, you can listen to my heart."

I lifted Diego onto the exam table and began his well-child exam, checking off the boxes of a head-to-toe assessment in my mind. At the end, I asked Diego to hop off the table so I could complete a brief musculoskeletal exam. I was almost ready to celebrate successful completion of the visit when I noticed something odd.

"Diego, can you do this?" I asked, demonstrating that I wanted him to lift both arms up over his head.

He nodded and stretched his right arm over his head.

"Good, but what about the other arm?"

He shook his head. "*Me duele*," he said. (It hurts.)

I should have noticed sooner, but at least I had picked up on it now. Diego had kept his left arm nearly motionless the whole time I had been in the room.

I reached out and gently tried to lift his arm, but he pushed me away with his right hand, saying "No, no!" Tears came to his eyes.

I turned to his mother. "His left arm—he can't move it. Did he injure it?" I asked in Spanish.

"*Sí,*" she said. "*Hace tres días.*" (Three days ago.)

Diego's mom explained he had fallen out of a swing at the playground and didn't want to move his arm ever since. He didn't have insurance—and she didn't have "papers" because the family was undocumented—so they hadn't gone to the emergency room. She thought maybe he was getting better.

I ran my hand along Diego's upper arm, under the sleeve of the Cookie Monster T-shirt. His arm seemed okay, but he winced when I poked on the front of his shoulder and collarbone.

"It's okay," I said, patting him on the back a couple of times and turning back to his mom. I wanted to ask why she hadn't told me about his arm, but I pushed aside my frustration. She had bigger worries. This woman, I discovered, had been deserted by the kids' father. She couldn't be making much more than minimum wage, if that. Her family was in Mexico, in a city ravaged by violence. She had few connections and only a couple of friends in Austin. Parenting a four-year-old was tough, even in ideal circumstances. Raising a teenager probably wasn't easy either. She couldn't keep track of everything.

"We need to do an x-ray. I think Diego has a broken shoulder," I said. "You'll need to go get the x-ray for him as soon as you leave here. My assistant will give you instructions. Can you do that?"

She nodded with a sad, resigned expression. I stepped out of the room to make sure Sara Maria was preparing Diego's vaccines and to order the shoulder x-ray, which would be discounted, though not free. I hated to add to this family's financial hardship, but I didn't see a way around it. Then I stepped back in to talk with Diego's fourteen-year-old sister.

Esperanza was the picture of an apathetic teenager. Her thick mascara and dark eyeliner made her look almost ghoulish. She refused to look at me, continuing to fiddle with her fingernails, one of which she seemed particularly interested in. She answered my questions by shrugging her shoulders. When she did speak, I could barely hear her.

"So, what high school will you go to next year?" I asked.

"Not going," she said, almost imperceptibly.

"What's that? It sounded like maybe you said you're not going to high school?"

"I'm not," she mumbled, just slightly louder this time.

"Why not?"

She shrugged her shoulders.

"Do you have any plans?" I asked.

Nothing. I looked at her mom, who mirrored her daughter's shrug. "What can I do?" she seemed to say.

"Well, is that okay with you?" I asked her mom, struggling a little with my Spanish. I think I may actually have said something like, "Does that seem well to you?"

"I can't make her go to school," she replied, shrugging again.

"You can tell her she *has* to go to school. You are her mother!" I said, stumbling again with my Spanish, trying to retain a hint of composure, even as my voice rose.

My reaction was immature, uncontrolled. I knew better.

Esperanza's mom gave a little half smile and shook her head.

I reeled my emotions back in. I had not yet parented a teenager. I remembered my list of Things I Used to Criticize but Now Understand. Small at first—screen time for kids under four and inflexible nap schedules—it now included leashes for children, boarding school, and boob jobs. I expected further additions as my kids grew older.

That's the thing about being a parent. Your kids challenge you and expand you as well. They offer profound new insights and perspectives. They teach you more about yourself while revealing who they are. I now did things I never thought I'd do. And I would *not* have found it helpful if someone had said to me, "Just tell Clara she *has* to go to sleep. You're her mother!"

"I'd like to talk to Esperanza alone for a minute. We can go to another room, and you can wait here with Diego. The medical assistant will bring his vaccines," I said, opening the door and motioning for Esperanza to follow me.

Once inside the exam room across the hall, I sat down on a stool across from Esperanza to begin a conversation about the Most Embarrassing Subjects that is a part of the standard annual checkup for teenagers. In her case, it would be the "Sex, Drugs, and How 'bout Staying in School?" talk.

"So, I wanted to give you an opportunity to talk to me privately in case you have any concerns or questions you don't want to discuss in front of your mom," I said, reciting my standard opening lines. "Do you have anything you'd like to talk about?"

Esperanza just looked at the floor. *Big surprise.*

I paused for a few seconds, letting my own gaze fall. The air in the exam room seemed too warm for early January. I'd have to ask Sara Maria or Kim to check the heat. But my discomfort wasn't just because of the temperature. I was dreading the next part of our conversation. I took a deep breath and looked back at Esperanza.

"So, if you don't have any questions for me, I have a couple more things to ask you," I said, feeling like I was reading from a script that still felt awkward, despite years of practice. I started with the more benign questions—How are things at school and home?—then moved on to the questions about smoking, alcohol, and drug use. She denied using substances, and she muttered something like "I'll think about it" when I urged her to stay in school, to make it a goal to graduate.

Still, the whole conversation felt pointless. I was doing this so I could check off more boxes to show I had asked the right questions—the questions I was trained to ask in any teen wellness visit. But even as I went through the motions, I was concerned about this kid. I really did care. This girl's life had been rough, unstable, full of struggle and loss. I didn't want the same for her future.

"So, one more thing—one thing that comes up for some kids in middle school is that some kids start to have boyfriends and girlfriends. . . . Some kids start having sex." I paused, wondering how I could say this in a less clumsy way. She continued to stare at the floor.

"Do you have a boyfriend?" I asked. Looking back, I realize I was making assumptions about her sexual orientation. I should have asked in a more neutral way. But Esperanza answered me.

"Used to," she said, looking up for a second before fixating again on the floor.

"Have you had sex?"

"Yeah, a long time ago."

"When was the last time?" I asked.

"I don't know . . . a week ago?"

A week ago. Right. Too long ago to consider a morning-after pill, too soon for a pregnancy test.

Esperanza went on to tell me that her mom already knew about her sexual activity. When I queried her mom about it a few minutes later, she answered with the same shrug. Her helplessness frustrated me, but her life was devoid of the kinds of real choices I took for granted. Her resignation was acceptance, an essential coping strategy, given her impossible circumstances.

We talked for a few more minutes, and I handed Esperanza a packet of information on contraceptive options since she didn't want to start birth control that day.

"*Gracias, Doctora*," her mom said. "*Gracias por hablar con no-sotros.*" (Thanks for talking with us.)

I looked at her, surprised. "*Con mucho gusto*," I said. "*Nos vemos pronto.*" (See you soon.)

As I finished writing notes from their appointments, I thought of Esperanza and Diego's mom's expression of thanks, hoping I might be able to help this family. I couldn't repair all that had gone wrong for them. I had to be aware of my limitations and temper my frustration that I couldn't get the mom a better job, health insurance for the family, and a safe place to live, surrounded by friends, where they could thrive. I couldn't stop the racism, xenophobia, and anti-immigrant sentiments that must have made their lives that much harder. I had to make my peace with knowing what was needed and being unable to make it happen. But perhaps I could find some shred of strength, some little bit of good that we could build on.

"You can't fix everyone; it's not your job to save the world," Don reminded me often. But over time, maybe we could make progress— Diego's broken clavicle would heal, and Esperanza could be referred to a counselor and supported to stay in school. I would see them back in a couple of days to review Diego's x-ray and discuss birth control options in more detail with Esperanza and her mom.

Leaving the clinic that day, I reflected on my afternoon. I had seen five or six patients, numbers that were simply awful by most standards. But, I told myself, I have to start back slowly, and hopefully I helped those patients. I had discovered Diego's injury, talked to Esperanza about contraception, and provided vaccines to both. It wasn't enough. It never felt like enough. But it was a privilege to be able to try, to be granted rare access to the lives of those I'd never meet otherwise, to support them, to learn from them. I wouldn't be a member of Congress like my dad or a Nobel laureate, but at least I had the interesting challenge of helping those most in need and serving my community.

CHAPTER 12:

Out of Control

January 2010

"You're going to relapse at some point. Nearly everyone does—it's almost certain," Dr. Reynard told me at my next neurology appointment. "We just don't know when."

Don took my hand as we processed this news. Despite the glossy advertisements for various MS wonder drugs on the exam room bookshelf, Dr. Reynard's proclamation wasn't a surprise. It was consistent with the little I'd allowed myself to read since my diagnosis. (Don and I still were avoiding articles on MS out of self-preservation.) I also knew that the form my relapse would take was unknown: I could lose my mobility, dexterity, or bladder control. I could develop any combination of incapacitating fatigue, heat intolerance, pain, depression, or cognitive dysfunction. I could lose my vision, at least temporarily, maybe permanently. MS didn't follow a pattern; it was unpredictable.

It could sit idly by and let me live my life, or it could attack like an army, explode like a Texas thunderstorm.

"So what will cause me to relapse?" I asked.

"We don't know what causes disease progression any more than we know what causes MS," Dr. Reynard said. "There are theories, of course. Heat, fatigue, stress? Those can provoke pseudorelapses—an increase in prior symptoms—but they won't cause a true relapse with new demyelination." He was referring to the nerve damage that characterizes MS, the destruction of myelin, the coating around nerve cells, which acts as a sort of insulation.

"I kind of figured. So, what can I do?"

"Apart from the usual healthy habits I'm sure you're familiar with, you can't do anything," he said.

That was a new one. *You can't do anything.* I didn't quite know what to think.

I vacillated between relief and frustration. The control freak in me was furious that I couldn't stop my current symptoms or keep MS from getting worse. I was already doing all the "usual healthy habits." I had kind of wanted Dr. Reynard to say that yes, ten hours of sleep every day was key to preventing disease progression. Or even a detailed, impossible-to-follow, anti-inflammatory diet; aromatherapy with lavender oil; handstands and cartwheels; magnets and reflexology; fresh-squeezed cranberry juice; antigravity chambers. Something. Anything.

Yet the fact that MS was out of my control was strangely comforting. I was the passenger, not the driver—and it's usually easier to be the passenger. It relieved me of responsibility. If things got worse, it wouldn't be my fault. It would be a long time before I really understood what it meant to give up control—or some of it, anyway—but there, in the doctor's office, in the midst of all that news of my inevitable demise, I felt myself . . . not relax, but loosen my grip on the steering wheel. Perhaps there was a shift in the set of my shoulders, a sense that I could even try to go with the flow.

I also was fortunate that so far I seemed to have the more common form, called "relapsing, remitting." This type of multiple sclerosis, which affects about 85 percent of MS patients, is characterized by periods of worsening symptoms or exacerbations that then get better, or remit, over time. Although I might accumulate disability, as we doctors would say, meaning I might start to lose certain skills and functions like strength or balance, I could also expect improvement between symptomatic periods. The frequency and severity of exacerbations, though, were variable and unpredictable. And I could someday, like many MS patients, end up with the secondary progressive form of the disease, which is difficult to stop and to treat.

"I guess it's just hard to believe that I'm powerless," I finally said.

"Well, that's not completely true," he said. "You can take your medicine. You should do all the stuff anyone should to be healthy: eat a good diet, stay active, don't smoke. All of that's very important. And, of course, avoid too much stress."

Stress. That was my problem. I could do everything else—the health food, exercise, medicines. I could go to yoga and avoid getting overheated. Stress, though, was ingrained, inevitable.

I wasn't alone. Even before the emergence of COVID-19, nearly one-third of Americans reported "extreme stress." Three-quarters of us experienced physical symptoms of stress, such as fatigue, headache, or upset stomach.[1] The pandemic exacerbated the problem. According to a survey in early 2021, a whopping 84 percent of adults reported feeling at least one emotion linked to prolonged stress in the prior two weeks, most commonly anxiety, sadness, and anger.[2] Most of my patients didn't talk about stress explicitly. They didn't have the luxury of considering stress to be a byproduct of a particular situation or set of circumstances. It was just how they felt, and they demonstrated it with their tears, pain, and panic attacks. Helping them find that connection was part of my role.

For me, stress was a fuel that kept me going even while wearing me down. I didn't think it was making me sick, exactly, but it couldn't be helping. When Dr. Reynard's advice was echoed by others living with MS whom I met in the weeks after my diagnosis, I realized reducing stress had to be a top priority.

Don and I started to gather tips and advice through our growing connection to the MS community—and we were amazed by the number of connections there were. Suddenly, everyone had a friend or a spouse or a sibling with MS. Many were in good health, happy to share their stories, and provide encouragement. Stress management was a common challenge.

Sally had been diagnosed with MS in her early twenties, long before those expensive new medications were available. According to Dr. Reynard, the prevailing sentiment at that time among neurologists was "Diagnose and *adiós*," meaning that once the doctor figured out someone had MS, they could say goodbye because there was nothing else they could do. However, Don had worked with Sally for years at the hospital, and until she heard about me and approached him, he had never known she had MS. She looked like she could be the star of a vitamin commercial, not someone with fuzzy white spots on her MRI.

Now in her fifties, Sally had been lucky. "I am able to lead a pretty normal life," she told Don and me when we went to talk to her. "I work full-time. I love my job, getting to work with kids every day.

"I've relapsed, sure," she continued. "Once I took my kids to Schlitterbahn—the water park. I knew I would pay for it later—the noise, the crowds, the heat. But it was worth it."

Such stories of system overload were becoming more familiar. Heat, in particular, was known to aggravate MS symptoms. But each person was different. I would have to figure out my own triggers.

Sally described a relapse when she hadn't been able to walk for two months. But she had managed to fully recover each time her MS flared. Stress reduction—and to my delight, a vegetarian diet—were part of her stay-healthy strategy.

"I have to conserve my energy," she said. "My husband has to help out more—picking up things around the house, that sort of thing."

"I'm liking the sound of this advice." I looked at Don.

"I don't remember agreeing to this meeting," he said, breaking into a smile.

We laughed. I lightly punched his upper arm. "Right," I said. "I dragged you here. Sally and I have a conspiracy going to get you to help more."

As much as I hated the million things getting out of place and cluttering my house, my stress reduction plan would involve far more than a renewed commitment from Don to clean up. I could barely manage my kids and the clinic before the diagnosis. Now I was also struggling with insomnia and having to give myself daily injections of my new medication. Don and I had so much going on that we could barely find a few child-free hours to spend together each month. I even forgot to pick up Ella from preschool one day.

For the first time in my life, I also missed a doctor's appointment. I was the no-show. At first, I was mortified. I knew what a no-show did to a doctor's schedule. I prided myself on being the reliable one.

"I'm so, so sorry. I promise you, I'm not that type of person," I said. "It will never happen again."

"What type of person?" the receptionist said, laughing. "It's okay. Sometimes life gets in the way."

On those rare occasions when I did get more caught up, when the downpour of concerns was reduced to a light shower, I would start searching for worries. I would focus on a minor faux pas: that phone call to a friend when I mistook her voice for her husband, addressing her by his name. Or I'd mentally reprimand myself, over and over, for my ridiculous attempt to bond with a young patient who was caught sneaking candy, by telling her I used to do the same thing (which wasn't even true). I felt unsettled if I didn't have an urgent, impossible task about to crush me—like I'd left the house without my shoes or forgotten something I wanted to say. My natural state was to be super-saturated with anxiety, and I would do whatever I could to get back to that baseline. Now the need to cut back on stress, on the off chance that it might help, made me even more stressed.

I hadn't exactly chosen a low-key profession. My patients danced from one crisis to the next, struggling with insurmountable financial as well as medical problems. Many faced both blatant and more subtle racism, impacting their access to care, to resources, to justice itself. Some of my patients from Del Valle, an impoverished and largely Hispanic community on the eastern edge of Austin, shopped for food at convenience stores for lack of a decent grocery store in their part of town. Others, in the midst of a health crisis, would be dismissed by the emergency room without a reasonable workup. I didn't know for sure, but I wondered if their disheveled appearance, their inability to advocate for themselves, maybe even their skin color impaired their ability to get the care and services they needed. I knew not to take on their problems as my own. But there's something about being in the room with these issues: insurmountable, never-ending, an avalanche, wanting to help and not knowing how. . . .

At the time I didn't know the term "moral distress," but it's since been used to describe the all-too-familiar situation when a doctor's ethical values collide with societal or institutional restrictions. On a gut level, I understood the concept long before it was given a name. I faced moral distress when I needed to refer my patient to a rheumatologist for suspected lupus, but I knew she'd never be able to afford it. Or when I talked to a single mom of four little kids about the need to do the impossible: stick to a regular sleep schedule and reduce stress to help her migraines.

As physicians, we are expected to be healers. But in a society plagued by prejudice, institutional racism, and inequality, we are forever running into obstacles when we try to help our patients— impossibly expensive medications, onerous program eligibility requirements for discounted care, medical records that are lost in transit. It's worse if our patients lack resources, an education, and basic skills, if they can't read or walk well or speak English. The United States is the only high-income country that doesn't provide universal coverage, despite spending far more on health care than any other nation. Tens of thousands of people die every year as a result of being uninsured. We physicians live with a deep frustration and sadness when we can't do what really needs to be done for those who come to us for help.

For me, the other responsibilities of managing a clinic—budget meetings, staff evaluations, scheduling decisions—also felt overwhelming. When I wasn't seeing patients, I was meeting with foundations that provided financial support, writing grant reports, reviewing productivity expectations, and teaching students who rotated through the clinic. It never stopped.

But the stress of work was nothing compared to problem number two: the kids. In comparison, going to work was easy.

"So, what do you think? Does stress cause MS symptoms to get worse? Can it cause a relapse?" I asked another one of my new friends with MS—a fellow physician who had diagnosed himself when he woke up completely numb and unable to walk seven years earlier.

He chuckled. "If you're not stressed, you're dead," he said. "Life is stressful. And you've got two kids—what, two and four? Well, that's just two nervous breakdowns waiting to happen."

Exactly.

My kids were a reason to get up every morning. Watching them discover the world was an unparalleled joy. I loved introducing them to my favorite places and things—the peacocks at Mayfield Park, the frigid water at Barton Springs, Mexican vanilla ice cream at Amy's. We spun under the Zilker Christmas Tree and played in the sand at the Austin City Limits Music Festival. We washed our dog, Mocha, and made pancakes on Sunday mornings.

And they were a reason not to get up. The screaming, clinging, complaining were ceaseless. Even the fun stuff was exhausting: the search for the next creative art project or kid-friendly recipe, planning the next holiday or vacation. When I walked in the door after a demanding day, Clara and Ella pounced on me. They were . . . like kittens attacking a ball of yarn? No, more like baby vultures devouring roadkill. At work I heard, "Doctor, I don't have time to exercise. That medicine you gave me doesn't work. Can't you do something else to fix me?" At home, it was "Mommy, Mommy, Mommm! I need a snack! I want an apple . . . with the peel cut off. . . . Mom! Why did you cut off the peel?"

Taking care of myself while attending to the needs of two whole little people was an impossible balance before MS. My medical training had taught me to ignore my own needs: thirty-six-hour shifts with almost no sleep, working weekends and holidays, skipping meals to admit patients to the hospital. The patient always comes first. Then, once I had Ella and Clara, my kids had to come first, maybe even before the patient, definitely before me. MS threw the hierarchy of needs into disarray. Suddenly I had to take care of myself, because if I didn't, the patients and the kids would suffer. I had to lower my expectations and relinquish some independence. I had to get more help. A lot more help.

When I was first diagnosed with MS, I told people immediately. I called my coworkers from the car on the drive home after the MRI. I told my running pal, Jess, in the parking lot during morning drop-off at our kids' preschool. I called Laura, Hannah, Marcia, and other friends and family over the next few days.

"Do you really want to do that?" asked my mom, ever practical and protective. "You know, this is considered a disability. People may not look at you the same way."

I thought about it and decided, yes, I wanted to tell people. I'm not a secretive person, and I realized I would be more stressed hiding big news from friends. Don—my usually introverted husband—felt the same way, to my relief.

I've never regretted being open about MS. Secrets can take on a life of their own. They take energy. They feed that sense of shame we feel when we can't maintain an impossible image of ourselves living the perfect life—the happy posts on social media, the smiles, the reassurances we provide whenever someone asks, "How are you?"

Some people who become ill feel they have to hide their condition from others, for fear of losing a job, a promotion, or even a friend. I've had patients—like some with PTSD or HIV—who suffer alone because the stigma is too much. "My family wouldn't understand if I tell them I'm depressed. They'll just tell me I'm weak," some have said. I've encouraged them to find someone to talk to—a cousin, a neighbor, a pastor, a teacher. Even just one trusted friend can ease the burden. A chronic condition can feel heavy and lonely. By sharing mine, I hope to normalize it for others, to make it okay to be authentic and vulnerable. I know not everyone is able to do the same.

For the friends I couldn't contact directly, I sent an e-mail:

"I am so sorry for the mass mailing, and I really feel bad for sharing major news via e-mail. Please know that I wish I could call each of you, but I'm overwhelmed and exhausted, so I'm resorting to my less-than-favorite form of communication. . . ."

I went on to share that I had MS. "That's a whole lot better than having a brain tumor, which is what Don and I had been thinking the night before the MRI, but of course it's not good news either. . . . We're just taking it one step at a time for now, and I'm hopeful that I'll be able to continue most of my usual activities once I get over the acute 'flare' I'm experiencing now."

It was paradoxically the same as and completely different than announcing an engagement or a pregnancy. It was big. It was life changing. And I was breaking some unwritten rules by being so open, maybe even creating fear or disappointment for those who received my message. I didn't want to burden anyone, not even with the feeling of obligation to respond, and I told them so. But they wrote back anyway, with beautiful notes of encouragement, thoughtful advice, offers to help.

"I wanted you to know how much I'm thinking about you," wrote one friend I didn't know particularly well. "And to tell you that we're here, in the neighborhood, and so available on short notice. . . . Consider us up for cooking or driving or anything else. Please don't hesitate."

As the visiting nurse set up my infusion of megadose IV steroids in the week after my diagnosis, one of my mom's best friends brought veggie burgers for dinner.

"I'll be back tomorrow with something from Texas French Bread," she said.

My sister arrived to play with Ella and Clara, give them a bath, and get them ready for bed. I lay on the couch next to an IV pole like an invalid—or maybe like a fairy-tale queen, since I just sat there surrounded by pillows and had everyone fussing over me.

Remembering this early support, I decided to reach out again. A part of me protested: I didn't want to annoy people or steal their free time. I didn't want them to think that I was weak or incapable of managing my kids and my life. But I knew that I did need help. I didn't have to try to do it all.

"I have an idea," I told Don a couple of evenings later, after reviewing his calendar and noting several more upcoming weekend and evening shifts.

"What's that?" he asked, glancing up from his crossword puzzle.

"You know how you've told me a bunch of times to get more help from the babysitter, like when you're working evenings and I'm alone with the kids?"

"Yeah, I still think you should do that," Don said.

"Well, okay, but I don't want to spend a lot of money. Plus, you know, I want to see the kids. I just get overwhelmed without any help, especially when I've been at work all day or if I'm dizzy," I said.

I explained to Don that I was going to start scheduling friends to come over in the evenings when he was at work and on weekends when my mom couldn't help. I also would get more help from a babysitter, on the weekends and in the mornings, at least a couple of days each week, to get us out the door. That day Clara, as usual, had refused to eat breakfast, wouldn't let me brush her hair, and chose mismatched clothes that looked ridiculous. I ended up late to my morning meeting.

With Don's encouragement, I sent e-mails to my sister and several friends with lists of days and evenings Don was working. I felt a little uneasy and hesitant—to be asking for, rather than offering, help—but I thought these evenings with friends and the kids could be fun for everyone. Lemonade from lemons. "Can you join us for dinner, bath time, and story time?"

My friends wrote back that they would be happy to help: Anita would bring stew one Thursday, Terin would come build forts with us and stay for dinner, Cathy would help me cook another night and take the kids for three hours on Saturday. Although my mom kept the kids for long stretches whenever she was in town on the weekends, she lived in Washington, DC, and wasn't always around. I lined up sitters for those weekends so that I could escape to the gym or a nearby café. I enlisted a helper to come in the mornings, just for an hour or two, so I could go on a short run and have support getting the kids ready for school.

And Don—whose concern and attention had stunned me in those first weeks after my diagnosis—had recovered from Christmas, and he did help more. He'd straighten up the house on his days off. Our division of labor drifted toward true equality. And when he was home in the evenings, he often would put the kids to bed to give me a break.

Most spectacularly, when it came to Clara's middle-of-the-night awakenings, I was the Default Parent No More. We trained her: "When you have growing pains or need water or have a nightmare, wake up Dad, if you must. Let Mom sleep."

At first, Clara didn't understand. She would creep up to my side of the bed. "Mom, I can't sleep. . . . Mom?"

"Clara. *Why?* Why are you waking me up?" I would say. I couldn't *not* be grouchy. I couldn't even be fake calm.

"I can't sleep."

Sigh. "Really? You're waking me up again. For that? What am I supposed to do?"

"I want to sleep in here."

"Uh, no."

"I don't like my bed."

On and on we'd go.

But Don intercepted. "Come here, Clara. You can lie with me for a minute, and then you have to go back to bed."

Gradually I trained myself to stay calm when I diverted Clara to Don during these middle-of-the-night interruptions. My maternal instinct was to control every interaction with the kids, but I resisted the urge and allowed myself to trust Don, even if he handled the situation differently than I would.

Clara learned to comply. Don was nicer in the middle of the night. He could fall back asleep more easily. To my delight, after a few interrupted nights, I really didn't have to tend to her anymore.

The image of the smooshed caterpillar as a symbol of our marriage was replaced by something different: a mountain, perhaps. Yes, I liked

CHAPTER 13:

Diseases That Really Suck

October 1995, January 2010

I nearly failed cell biology and histology. All first-year medical students were required to take this class—CBH, we called it—which focused on the intricacies, form, and function of the different kinds of cells. We learned about all systems of the body at the microscopic level. Our textbook devoted entire chapters to "The Nucleus" and "Cytoplasm and Organelles." We studied dynein, the Golgi apparatus, microtubules—words and concepts that meant nothing to most of us before or after that sixteen-week period of our lives.

The only thing good about the class was the professor. Dr. Frank Kretzer's enthusiasm about cells was almost contagious. He pranced around the lecture hall, as animated as a little kid in a toy store. He was delighted by the regenerative properties of epithelial tissues. He was fascinated by transcription factors and helicases. He couldn't get enough of the immune system. "And look at these neutrophils! They are the first responders, racing to stop an infection, attacking the threat, using phagocytosis, degranulation, reactive oxygen species— positively elegant!" he proclaimed.

Even with a talented instructor, I struggled. I wanted to be interested, to *want* to learn the material. But to me, reading the ingredients of a tube of toothpaste would have been better than studying my CBH textbook. When I scored a "marginal pass" on midsemester exams, I got nervous. I was at risk of failing a class for the first time in my life. But Dr. Kretzer didn't want anyone to fail. He invited me to join a series of extra tutoring sessions: remedial CBH. That's where I found my study partner, Julia.

Together, Julia and I helped each other pass the class. We attended remedial CBH two evenings a week, in a small room on an upper floor of the medical school. The fluorescent lights bounced off the dark windows that lined one wall, and Dr. Kretzer stood near the front, next to a slide projector, bursting with excitement to tell us more about mitochondria and ribosomes. Seven or eight other first-year medical students joined us for those sessions, all of us feeling both embarrassed to be there and grateful for the extra help. Julia and I also met on other nights, quizzing each other on the differences between desmin, vimentin, and cytokeratin—mysterious terms for what our cell biology professor told us were the "intermediate filaments" of various body parts—and inventing funny mnemonics to remember new words and definitions. We continued to study together in the subsequent months as we moved on from classes about normal body mechanics and functions to focus on everything that can go wrong. While we could never muster the same enthusiasm for our studies that Dr. Kretzer exhibited for cells, we did find creative ways to absorb the massive amount of material required.

To help us remember rare conditions and obscure infections, for instance, we sometimes found ourselves in an animated debate about the worst of the Diseases That Really Suck.

"Leishmaniasis—a rare life-threatening parasitic infection spread by sandflies," Julia reviewed, tugging at her baseball cap. "Dude, this one *really* sucks. One form of it causes gross skin sores that can take years to heal and lead to horrible scars. It can also cause internal organ damage, fever, and anemia."

"I don't know. I mean, it sounds pretty bad, but, like, a glioblastoma brain tumor seems worse. Or rabies! Definitely rabies is worse," I said.

"Rabies. Geez. Okay, yeah, that's worse. But that's a virus. It's not on the test this week."

"I know. I'm just saying there are worse things."

"Yeah, but let's get through the parasites."

I looked down at my notes. I had created a chart, with almost microscopic handwriting, listing all the parasites we were expected to know. I had thought writing it all down might help me remember, though most of the material wouldn't stick easily.

"Okay. What about Strongyloides stercoralis? That one's even found in Texas," I said.

"So that's the threadworm, right? And yeah, it's bad in immunosuppressed people, but most people don't have symptoms."

"If you're immunosuppressed it really sucks, though," I said. "Like, it can start off with these vague abdominal symptoms, and you don't think it's a big deal, but then it spreads, and you can get meningitis and sepsis."

"For the average person, Leishmaniasis sounds worse."

As we bantered about these terrible, often life-ending diseases, we missed a key point, one that took me years to grasp fully: The Diseases That Really Suck are not determined so much by the diagnosis but rather the context, the resources, whether family and friends will call and drop by. I've befriended people with progressive multiple sclerosis—the less common and more serious form of MS that is harder to treat. Some use wheelchairs. Some have worsening symptoms and disability despite the best new treatment options. But their lives are rich and full because of their connections, their will to fight and stay active, their commitment to reach outside themselves to help others, despite their limitations.

As Don started to remind me after the discovery of white spots on my MRI, we were lucky. In medical school I had Dr. Kretzer and Julia to help me pass a difficult class. Now, as I faced a new challenge, I had family nearby. I had health insurance. I had friends who came to help me in the evenings. We could build on our "luck" by nurturing those friendships, by seeking new connections, perhaps in the MS community. Gratitude, not fear and resentment, should be our focus.

If only my patients had access to the same support.

Mauricio, debilitated after his electrical burns, had stopped coming to see me. I don't know what happened to him, but I think we somehow determined that he and his wife had returned to Mexico. He had been improving, and we were working to control his diabetes and prepare for another surgery to modify one of his skin grafts. But perhaps he decided to forgo further medical treatment, opting to be with his own support circle. I couldn't blame him and felt thankful to be spared such an agonizing choice.

We now know that the conditions in which we live, work, learn, and play—called "social determinants of health" (SDoH)—have a far greater impact on health than any medical treatment we can offer. Despite our obsession with developing and providing state-of-the-art therapies to cure disease, it's the social determinants—like access to housing and healthy food, transportation, and safe neighborhoods— that drive 80 to 90 percent of health outcomes on a population level.

People of color are more likely to struggle with basic resources that contribute to poor health outcomes. But they also face inequities that extend far beyond the more obvious financial divisions. I often took it for granted, but I knew that my race put me at a particular advantage. African Americans, Hispanics, and Native Americans suffer from higher rates of chronic disease than non-Hispanic whites. Although the gap between whites and Blacks has narrowed, African Americans face a shorter life expectancy, even after controlling for economic indicators. In recent years, for example, we've learned that maternal mortality rates in African American women are more than three times higher than for white women.[1] During much of the COVID-19 pandemic, people who were Black, Hispanic, or Native American got sick and died at far higher rates than white Americans, when accounting for age differences, largely due to increased poverty, occupational exposure, increased reliance on public transportation, and limited access to health care.[2] High rates of certain chronic conditions, like diabetes and heart problems, probably played a role as well. Long-standing biases in our health care system have meant that, in many cases, those who need the most help get the least.

Additionally, social isolation increases the risk of anxiety, depression, heart disease, stroke, dementia, and premature death from all causes.[3] So many of my patients suffered from a deep loneliness that I could never eradicate. Over the years I had coached many to ask for help, to think of their neighbors and friends who might drive them to an appointment or organize their medicines. Some had family who would rally around them, but others didn't know whom to ask. "Your friends want to help," I might say. But some of my patients didn't seem to have friends. Many had been uprooted so often they didn't have a chance to make connections. Others were isolated in their homes due to mobility issues, lack of transportation, or even fear.

Sometimes I fantasized about matchmaking: *Connie, Alejandra, and Rose Marie could be friends,* I thought. *They all seem lonely, yet they are nice people.* But patient confidentiality laws made that impossible. It was hard for me to imagine, but some people had virtually no one.

I have had to give bad news—sometimes far worse than an MS diagnosis—to countless patients. And sometimes I'm the only one offering support. My responsibility, in those cases, seemed to take on a new level of importance after my own illness. I now understood on a personal, intimate level that connections with others are critical not just to pass tests in medical school but to bounce back from a health crisis. Realizing this, I gave thanks for the life I was privileged to lead, even as I struggled to control my resentment of MS and my fury, on behalf of my patients, at the System That Really Sucks.

Before my diagnosis I wouldn't have thought to appreciate the fact that I could walk or write or drive. Without MS, I wouldn't have experienced the love and concern from family and friends that had meant so much and helped sustain me during those early days after my diagnosis. I wasn't sure yet, but maybe my Disease That Kind of Sucks could be an opportunity to realize a new level of gratitude and compassion and a renewed commitment to fight for those people who didn't have anyone else.

CHAPTER 14

Whac-A-Mole

February 2010

Faith was returning to the clinic for her asthma. I could hear her coughing from down the hall. The reason for her visit, listed on my afternoon schedule, was "ER follow-up." After resolving her unreasonable bill for the knee x-rays some months back, I had secured an appointment for her in the asthma clinic. But she was on a long waiting list to be seen. Meanwhile, she was bouncing in and out of the ER and sometimes getting admitted to the hospital.

"Sara Maria, I can't find the ER notes. Can you pull them up?" I asked.

"We don't have them. She went to a different hospital this time, and we can't get those records through the computer. I've sent a request, but we're still waiting for their fax," she said. "I can't call. They always put me on hold, and I'm in the middle of discharging a patient for Terri."

Serving as a primary care physician for hundreds of patients is like reading hundreds of books simultaneously and losing track of the plot in most of them. Before seeing a patient for a follow-up visit, I had to skim through her records to see where I was in that person's story. Now, because of the missing ER notes, I would have to review the chart with the most recent chapter missing. Faith would have to fill in the gaps and catch me up.

Another problem I faced, not limited to Faith, was that the electronic medical record (EMR)—always clunky and unintuitive—had just been "upgraded." The labs and medication lists were in different places, and I had to flip through multiple screens, scrolling up and down, searching for relevant information. Some of my notes seemed to have disappeared altogether. Other sections of the electronic chart were out of order.

Although they had been around for decades in a limited capacity, EMRs became increasingly widespread in the years after implementation of the Health Information Technology for Economic and Clinical Health (HITECH) Act in 2009. By 2021 nearly 90 percent of office-based physicians used EMRs.[1] Electronic records were touted as a solution to improve efficiency and reduce errors, but they continue to be a major source of physician dissatisfaction and burnout. The particular EMR my practice was required to use was a disappointment for all of us, especially me. "Disappointment," in fact, is a nice way of putting it. I felt a twinge of satisfaction a couple years later when I saw the type of EMR we had ranked last on a user-satisfaction survey.

At times I wondered if my ineptitude with the EMR was due to a personal deficiency. Not everyone had so much trouble. A friend at another clinic could tally twice as many patient visits as me, using the same system. How was that possible? What was wrong with me? I had never been fast seeing patients, but now I wondered if my MS was making things worse.

Cognitive dysfunction is one of the most common symptoms of MS. More than half of people with MS will develop it over time. It can manifest as memory problems, impaired attention and concentration, difficulty with planning and prioritizing, and impaired word-finding. Myelin, the substance coating nerve cells that is damaged in MS, acts as a sort of insulation to the neuron. It made perfect sense that my information processing would be slower without proper insulation, and I worried it was affecting my work, especially with the EMR.

Dizziness could also have been a factor, making it hard to click between screens to check the right boxes. The intensity and persistence of my dizziness had dissipated over time, but I still wasn't back to normal.

I was already twenty minutes behind when I opened the door to the exam room. Faith didn't look good. Her pulse and blood pressure were elevated; her weight was up four more pounds in just two weeks. The medicines she took to keep her lungs functioning made continued weight gain almost inevitable. Yet with each additional pound, her health deteriorated.

"Hey, Faith! How's it going?" I said, realizing how enthusiastic I sounded. *Too enthusiastic.* My patient was not in the mood to feign cheerfulness.

"Hi, Dr. [breath] Doggett," she struggled, wheezing and ending with a long cough.

"You don't look good," I said. "I had hoped the higher dose of steroids would stop this stubborn asthma attack."

"No, it hasn't helped at—" she interrupted herself again with a cough.

I was attempting to log onto the computer to pull up her electronic chart while trying to listen to her. Probably because of something to do with the upgrade, the computer wouldn't accept my password at first; then it asked me to change my password. I wanted to look at Faith, but I couldn't break away from the computer. Making eye contact would require me to pause, and I didn't have that time.

"Hang on. I'm so sorry, but the electronic medical record is giving me trouble today," I said. I was violating the rule that I had learned in an amusing EMR training video that had accompanied the upgrade: never say anything negative about the EMR in front of a patient. Instead of screaming, "This goddamn machine is a piece of shit and is ruining my life," I was supposed to emphasize the benefits of the EMR to the patients: "Look how we can see all of your labs together in one place!" or "I'm going to send this prescription electronically to your pharmacy right now and then print out a copy of your medication list. How cool is that?" But at that moment, those advantages were overshadowed by enormous inefficiencies. I couldn't do anything because I couldn't log onto the computer.

I glanced up. "Did Sara Maria get an oxygen saturation level on you?" I was referring to a test we use to assess for oxygen deprivation. Faith was well versed in this terminology.

"Yeah, it was 86 percent today," she replied, coughing again. Normal levels range from 95 to 100 percent, and values under 90 are considered low. Usually, Faith's oxygen saturation hovered around 92. Eighty-six percent was bad even for her. I tried selecting a new password, but it was apparently the same password I had used at some point in the past, and the EMR rejected it.

"I hate to say it, but I think we're going to have to send you back to the ER. It sounds like you need to be admitted to the hospital again." I rolled my stool toward her to listen to her lungs.

"I thought you'd say that," she said, her face red from the effort of breathing.

I regretted spending time reviewing her chart before the visit. None of it mattered now. She was too sick for me to treat her in the clinic. Her lungs were noisy with loud wheezing on both sides. She was in respiratory distress.

I left the room to get Sara Maria's help, but she was checking in my next patient. I called the ER to tell them that Faith would soon be on her way. Her husband would drive her.

Although I managed to log back onto the computer after a call to the help desk, I still couldn't figure out how to order the tests I needed for my next three patients. The upgrade had changed the process. Ordering a mammogram took seventeen mouse clicks but was doable. A thyroid ultrasound, used to assess an enlarged thyroid or a thyroid nodule, had to be ordered as a "neck" ultrasound. I only figured this out after searching and searching again for the thyroid test and finally asking Terri, who had called the help desk earlier after running into the same problem.

The EMR had more bugs than my compost bin. The chest x-ray order for elderly Mr. Sanchez stated he was pregnant. Every new note I wrote defaulted to state "Rectum 0.0 cm" on the physical exam. Terri laughed when the intake note for a well-baby checkup stated that the four-month-old infant had zero sexual partners and was not currently taking birth control. Other tests seemed to be missing completely, like the bone density test I often ordered to check for osteoporosis.

By the sixth patient, I was nearly in tears. I had tried to put Faith out of my mind, but I worried about her worsening asthma, our inability to make progress. I was trying to keep up with my notes and orders on all my patients, but I kept getting further behind. I knew people were waiting for me, yet I couldn't get the EMR—the new, "better" version of the EMR—to do what I needed.

My escalating rage and frustration brought back a memory of Ella. When she was two years old, Ella often had trouble going to sleep. One night, in the midst of a bedtime-induced tantrum, furious little Ella marched down the stairs from her room and slammed the large antique bookshelf in our hallway, knocking it over. She had astounded me with her strength and violent tendencies. It had crashed into the wall, leaving gaping holes in the sheetrock. Now I summoned adult-level restraint to keep from following her example and hurling my computer through the tall glass window next to my desk.

I had one more patient to see, but I couldn't find Sara Maria anywhere, and the patient needed to be escorted to a room. I knew she was helping Terri, but I needed her to help me. Kim was on the phone with the vaccine refrigerator company after a catastrophic malfunction caused us to lose thousands of dollars' worth of immunizations. I had to finish so that I could pick up the kids at preschool, and I finally decided to just bring the last patient back to the room myself.

I grabbed a piece of scratch paper for taking notes, having given up on the EMR, and marched up to the waiting room to call Sherry back.

Sherry, at least, was doing great. *Could something actually be going right?*

"Dr. Doggett, my headaches are gone. I can't believe it, but that medicine really works. I'm sleeping better, and—you're not going to believe it—I've lost weight!" she gushed as we walked down the hallway. I held up my hand for a high five, and she slapped it and climbed on the scale.

"Wow, Sherry! You've lost seven pounds. That'll really help your diabetes and your blood pressure. Way to go!" I said.

Since her diabetes diagnosis several months before, Sherry had proved herself to be one of my superstar patients. I had worried that she wouldn't be able to manage, but Sherry had rallied, taking her medications, reading up on a diabetic diet, and joining the YMCA. She had brought in a blood pressure log with neatly recorded weekly readings that were all in the normal range. We looked at her labs. Her diabetes was well controlled, too.

"Any problems with your meds?" I asked.

"A little bit at first. Just some upset stomach, but I'm fine now. I must've gotten used to it."

She was resilient, but why? I didn't know what made her embrace health while others stayed stuck in a pit of despair, inaction, and bad habits. What could she teach me so I could help my other patients . . . so I could help myself?

"Sherry, you've done so well in spite of all you've got going on," I said. "How did you do it?"

"You know, the diabetes diagnosis . . . It wasn't the worst thing," she said. "It's actually made me take better care of myself. I even got a new job with normal hours. It was wake-up call, I guess."

"I'm so glad you can see it that way," I said. "It's really kind of inspiring."

And it was. That silver lining. The shift in thinking, in perspective.

Maybe I didn't have to abandon my dreams. Perhaps my own chronic condition could even be a launchpad for positive change.

"I'm really grateful for all your help," she said, smiling. "You know, I just found out I'm getting private insurance at work. This will be my last visit with you."

Our clinic didn't take private insurance, which meant that Sherry couldn't come back. I was always happy for my patients who were able to come up with more options for themselves, but frequently the ones who got insurance were the people who took their medicines and followed my advice—the ones who helped me feel a sense of accomplishment. The people who brought in blood sugar records and updated medication lists were the same ones who got new jobs, managed to join a spouse's insurance plan, or searched online for reasonably priced self-insurance policies. Once insured, they could afford a wider range of medications and have access to specialty care and radiology services. An ER visit or even a hospitalization might not drain their bank accounts if they even had bank accounts.

The infuriating paradox remained: My patients who needed insurance the most were often the least likely to get it. They had language barriers, illiteracy, mental health problems. They were scared of getting deported and scared of the messy, apathetic health care system. They were too busy finding a new job or a new apartment, figuring out ways to pay the utilities bill or get a car fixed that they didn't have time to look after themselves, to think about luxuries like exercise, fresh fruits and vegetables, and insurance. They were intimidated by doctors who talked down to them or talked over their heads: "You've got albuminuria, so we need to start an ACE-inhibitor, but we'll need to watch out for hyperkalemia . . ." or "Your triglycerides are sky-high, and your HDL is low, so it looks like you've got metabolic syndrome. We should probably start a fibrate to prevent pancreatitis, and you've got to lower your BMI." More than anything, my uninsured patients were too buried in the day-to-day to look to the future.

But not Sherry. She had beaten the odds.

"Oh, that's great—great you got insurance, I mean," I told her. "I'll miss taking care of you though." I refilled her blood pressure medicine and gave her a list of doctors I could recommend in the private insurance world. When I said goodbye, I felt like a teacher bidding farewell to a graduating student. Then I trudged back to my office to transcribe my handwritten notes into the EMR.

The EMR upgrade was supposed to be an improvement over the old system, but it wasn't. One colleague called it a "downgrade," and I agreed. It looked and felt different, but not better. I was relieved to learn that I wasn't alone in my struggle when a physician from an affiliated clinic e-mailed an example of one of his EMR notes after the upgrade. He called it "Master Document Stuttering."

"How's this for readability, readability, readability?" he wrote.

"Onset: 6 Month(s) ago. # Stools/day: 4. The patient describes it as foul odor, loose, watery, brown, green, foul odor, loose, watery and br The problem is worse. Relieving factors include Imodium, Imodium, Imodium, and Imodium. Associated symptoms include cramping, weight loss, cramping, weight loss, cramping, weight loss, cramping and weight loss. Additional information: no family history of colon cancer, no family history of Crohns/ Colitis, nightsweats, no family history of colon cancer, no family history of Crohns/Colitis, nightsweats and no family history of c."

He concluded, "If these records are ever sent to another facility, we'll be a laughing stock, laughing stock, laughing stock."

While I felt some validation when I read my colleague's e-mail, I was discouraged that we'd never meet our goals for productivity—the number of patient visits. I had hoped once we worked out the kinks, the EMR would improve our workflow. Alas, it was not to be.

I drove home on a Friday afternoon, reviewing my week and wondering how I would have the nerve to go back on Monday. Productivity aside, our clinic mini audit had just revealed multiple deficiencies:

no policy to deal with chemical spills, an expired fire extinguisher, no plan for regular equipment inspections. Who knew these things were supposed to be done? I didn't. We'd also detected a weird stink from the ceiling, and the building manager still hadn't sent the guy charged with investigating such mysteries.

And I had just had to tell a patient, a man in his late forties, that he was dying of metastatic lung cancer.

The humdrum details of clinic management, while important, clashed with the real catastrophes. Everything was happening at once, with no time to give each task the perspective and weight it deserved, no time for careful consideration or proper prioritizing.

Clara awoke twice that night, and though Don took care of her need for a cold glass of water and soothed the ache in her knee, I couldn't go back to sleep. I was trying to be grateful—for Don, for my parents and sister, for my friends who came to help in the evenings— but any real feeling of gratitude was relegated to the shadows. I lay there perseverating on my failure as a clinic director and embarrassing inefficiency as a doctor. MS made me feel powerless. I was now Less Likely to Succeed. Even if I adjusted our schedules, hired new staff, and became an EMR whiz, I couldn't cure poverty or fix our broken health care system.

I used to think I was good at my job. I had helped take care of Marvin, Faith, Amber, and Diego. I had convinced foundations to provide grants to the clinic. I had hired Kim and Sara Maria and others, building a team that often felt like a family. I used to think I had mastered wielding the mallet in a crazy game of Whac-A-Mole, attacking each new challenge with fervor and finesse. But now I didn't think we could ever meet our productivity goals. Every month, I sighed with resigned hopelessness when I got the tally of patient encounters: thirty-eight visits below goal one month, twenty-seven short the next. Everything seemed to be falling through the cracks. I could only see the deficiencies: the missing policies, the broken vaccine refrigerator, the stink in the ceiling. I was defective—brain damaged, in fact. Now I had become the little head in the game that keeps popping up again and again only to get smacked.

CHAPTER 15:

The Waiting Place

March 2010

The typical spring weather had returned. I took the kids to the downtown library after work to avoid a sticky, rainy afternoon at home. Afraid of another post office incident, I had avoided outings for months, but now Clara was older. I told myself it would be easier.

Ella seemed to have recovered from her morning crisis: no acceptable outfits to wear to preschool. I was downstairs getting breakfast for Clara and lamenting that my five-year-old had better fashion sense than I did.

"I hope Ella will settle down and come downstairs," I said to Clara, who was on her best behavior in the face of her sister's tantrum.

Ella overheard me, and with the appropriate volume and force of a conversation during a Metallica concert, she screamed, "I'm settling down!!!"

But she did seem calm and happy as we pulled into the parking lot.

I handed the girls matching blue bags from my mom—"for getting books at the library." We headed back, past the fiction section and rows of computers, to the children's section. I liked this part of the library best, with its big windows, cheerful rugs, and happy memories from my own childhood. Clara started grabbing books, trying to stuff some in her library bag, and knocking others to the floor. She was like a TV game show contestant, racing to fit as much in the shopping cart as possible.

"Mommy, I need help!" Ella said.

I gave myself a quick pep talk: *I can do this. Women and men come here with five kids and make it work. It's better to be here than holed up at home.*

"Clara, we can't take everything. Let's pick your six favorites." Then I turned to Ella. "Are you wanting to find Fancy Nancy like we talked about?"

"Yes!" Ella said.

"Well, you are five years old now, and I think you can go all by yourself to ask that nice librarian over there for help," I said, bracing myself for renewed whining.

But she surprised me. "Okay," she said, and she walked over to the librarian—an older woman who smiled at Ella and asked, "How can I help you, young lady?"

"I want to find Fancy Nancy, please."

"Right over here," the librarian said, stepping out from behind the desk to show Ella a row of books near one of the floor-to-ceiling windows. With Ella occupied, I could give Clara my full attention.

I was trying to reframe my feelings about Clara's behavior. She was "adventurous and inquisitive," not "destructive and messy."

At home, Clara would pull out Kleenex, put the empty boxes on her feet, and walk around the house. "I have new shoes!" she'd squeal. She spilled new bottles of bubbles. She ate tempura paint and painted everything except the paper. She discovered my mascara and smeared it all over her hands and face. She went through my mom's purse and took her credit card, which I found in a Hello Kitty box a couple days later. When she pulled the seat off her little potty and put it over her head like a necklace, she smiled and asked, "I'm a piece of work?" I assured her she was.

Clara's constant demands for me to build forts and do the alphabet house puzzle collided head-on with my need for space—to cope with dizziness, to rest, to just chill out. But at the library, I tried to follow her lead and let her put eight books in the bag, including two unseasonal Christmas books.

Ella came back with three Fancy Nancy books and two others with colorful pictures that she had noticed on display on top of one of the shelves. We walked back to the front of the library to check out.

"Mommy, can I get some water?" Ella asked as we passed the water fountain.

"Sure, just try not to touch your mouth directly to the place where the water comes out," I answered, lifting up Clara and joining the checkout line.

"Down!" Clara commanded. "I get water?"

"Okay, Clara, but then come right back here," I said as Clara ran to join her sister. Ella was carefully drinking to avoid touching the spout with her mouth.

Clara waited for a few seconds, but she wanted a turn. She had the patience of, well, a two-year-old. Ella was taking too long! Instead of pushing Ella out of the way as I expected, or shouting at her to move, she reached for either side of Ella's denim skirt, the one with the flowery ruffles. Ella continued to drink, oblivious. Gripping hard, Clara yanked the skirt down to Ella's ankles. I watched with a mix of horror and amusement as Ella stopped drinking water, noted that she was standing in the library in her underwear, and pulled up her skirt. Without a word to Clara, she moved out of the way, and Clara took her turn at the water fountain.

Well, that's one way to do it, I thought, handing over the books and Ella's library card to the checkout guy. I decided not to care what anyone else thought. Perhaps Clara made them laugh or gave them a funny story to tell. But it would be a while before I'd be brave enough to come back.

Clara's behavior that spring reinforced our belief that she, now nicknamed "Destructor," was the embodiment of entropy—that mysterious force leading all things to a state of disorder. But worse than the chaos she left in her path was Clara's continued failure—refusal— to sleep. Don or I would read her bedtime stories, cuddle with her, and tuck her into bed. It never, ever lasted. We thought that as doctors—a pediatrician and family physician, at that—we should know how to get our kid to sleep. Other parents asked *us* for advice about sleep; we were supposed to be experts. But Clara was a lost cause.

I counted myself lucky on the nights I could make it through teeth brushing and ten minutes of a show before Clara, who had recently learned to climb out of her crib, reemerged like Road Runner in a Looney Tunes cartoon. "My CD is broken," she might say. Or "I need water." As soon as that was resolved, she would be back with something else: "I have a boo-boo on my finger." It would be my turn to get a Band-Aid. She broke a so-called babyproofed door handle in three nights, so we put a lock on our own door. Clara's crying became familiar background music as Don and I made our way through Season 3 of *Lost* on DVD.

The toxic combination of sleep deprivation, MS worries, and my failure as a disciplinarian made me cringe when well-meaning elders cooed, "Oh, how fun to have two little girls! Don't blink. It goes by so fast!" "Are you kidding?" I wanted to say. "It doesn't go fast enough." And on the evenings Don worked, after my sister or helpful friend had gone home for the night, I would lie with Clara after two or three books. *How on earth am I going to get you to bed?*

When rationalization and bribery failed, I was sometimes reduced to the kind of parent I swore I'd never be. Enraged and panicked that stress and sleep deprivation would trigger an MS flare, I would shout almost as loud as Clara, "Oh my God! Please STOP CRYING!" I would plead with the desperation of someone fleeing a house fire. "Please, please, please, GO TO SLEEP!"

A page in my favorite Dr. Seuss book, *Oh, the Places You'll Go*, describes "the Waiting Place." In this "most useless place," people are "waiting for the fish to bite or waiting for wind to fly a kite or waiting around for Friday night or waiting, perhaps, for their Uncle Jake or a pot to boil, or a Better Break or a string of pearls, or a pair of pants or a wig with curls, or Another Chance. Everyone is just waiting."[1]

I could relate. I had been stuck in waiting rooms often since my MS symptoms started. I waited for Dr. Reynard, for labs, for the MRI. I waited for the insurance company to pick up the phone, for my medicine to be delivered, for results of all those tests.

Reading the book one night, I recognized a new waiting place. "Don, this is us!" I told him, flipping back to the page after putting

Clara to bed for the fourth time. "We're stuck in the Waiting Place, waiting for Clara to grow up. I know she's cute now, but I'm exhausted," I said. "Work plus MS plus Clara is just too much. I am *so* ready to be the parent of an older child."

CHAPTER 16:

Another Catch-22

March 2010

I didn't have to ask Andy, my new patient on Tuesday afternoon, why he had come to see me. A white man, nearly sixty, with a scruffy beard and a bald head, Andy jumped in right away, unprompted.

"I'm an alcoholic. I don't want to be, but I am," he said, after introducing himself. "That's why I'm here. I need to stop drinking."

I appreciated his candor. Many patients who are addicted to substances are evasive, in denial, or defensive. Not Andy. I asked him to tell me more about his drinking and what made him decide to quit.

"Where do I even start?" he asked. "I've been drinking as long as I can remember. And I've watched my world crumble because of it."

He recounted a tragic past: lost jobs, a divorce from the love of his life. "You know, I don't blame her for leaving. I couldn't be a proper husband." He had a sister who still checked on him sometimes, but she was busy raising three kids and lived in Temple, a small city sixty miles north of Austin.

"What's your situation now? Do you live alone?" I asked.

"Yeah," he said. "Well, except for my animals—two dogs and a cat. They keep an eye on me."

I smiled but felt a hint of concern. *No human housemates.* Still, "I'm glad you have some company. . . . So, I've got to ask, how much do you drink?"

"Well, whatever I can get," he said. "Probably two, three six-packs a day. Maybe a couple shots, too."

"A lot," I said.

"A lot," he agreed.

I asked Andy what he had tried in the past, and he gave me a list of what he described as "the usual," meaning cutting back, cold turkey, and rehab, once, years ago when he had insurance. He drew the line at Alcoholics Anonymous, though.

"I'm an atheist," he said. "All that shit in AA about God and a 'higher power'—it wasn't for me."

A lot of people get stuck on the "higher power" aspect of AA, but it doesn't have to be religious. AA groups of all types and flavors meet every day all over the world. While AA doesn't offer medical treatment to help people stop drinking, its well-known Twelve-Step program is one of the best, most effective ways for people struggling with alcohol addiction to achieve and maintain sobriety. Participation is free. I tried to get Andy to give AA another chance, but he was noncommittal.

"I'd do just about anything if I thought it'd help," he said. "I just don't think it would. Plus I need to detox. Isn't there some kind of inpatient program where I can go to sober up and figure things out?"

"Oh, I wish," I said. "I mean, if you were admitted to the hospital, they'd help you detox, but they won't admit you for the *purpose* of detox. They'd only do it if you happened to be there for something else." I was mad just saying it. The situation was ridiculous. For someone drinking as much as Andy, to quit suddenly was dangerous. But planned, controlled detox, done safely in an inpatient setting, was out of the question for an uninsured patient. It was a catch-22—the result of a lousy system designed for the benefit of . . . who? The hospital administrators? The chief financial officer? It reminded me of the rule for undocumented patients with kidney failure: They couldn't get dialysis in the United States unless it was an emergency, unless they were on the verge of dying without it. The people who most needed care couldn't get it until the last possible second.

"Yeah, that figures," he said.

Andy was uninsured. With no job, he had no real hope of getting insurance until he turned sixty-five and could sign up for Medicare. Because he owned a house and had a few other assets, he didn't qualify for the city's Medical Access Program, a safety-net option that provided limited health care coverage for low-income adults. Another catch-22. Andy belonged to what we used to call the "working poor," only he wasn't working—at least not in a consistent job. I don't know how he was able to afford his house, and I'm sure it worried him, too. Perhaps a relative took pity. It wasn't my place to probe. I didn't want to become entangled. I had to respect professional boundaries for my own safety and sanity, though sometimes they felt rigid, inhibiting my ability to connect with a fellow human being.

Even with insurance, getting Andy into an affordable detox program would have been difficult. I could only think of one option.

"I don't have a lot of experience with it, but I could help you detox as an outpatient," I said. I hated to even suggest it, because I knew it was risky, and I really didn't know how to do it.

"Really?" he asked. "I'm game."

Crap.

I'd prescribed medicines before for alcoholics struggling with withdrawal, but I'd never gotten someone down from three six-packs a day to nothing. Then again, I'd never had someone so ready to quit, ready to try "anything."

"Okay, well, it's not gonna be easy. I'll need to do some research to figure out the meds for you, but I know you're going to need to come back every day this week to see me. Could you do that?"

"I think so," he said.

I went back to my office and searched for information on medical regimens for safe outpatient detox. Bingo! I found an article in a family medicine journal: "Ambulatory Detoxification of Patients with Alcohol Dependence."

I was nervous. Abruptly stopping alcohol after years of heavy drinking could lead to serious withdrawal. The course of symptoms was unpredictable but might include tremors, sleep disturbance, nausea and vomiting, and anxiety. In some cases, there could be seizures, as well as the dreaded DTs: delirium tremens. More common in long-term heavy drinkers, DTs included severe mental status changes and hallucinations. In rare cases, withdrawal would lead to death.

Because the stakes are high, most people who aren't well supported by friends or family or who have certain other medical problems shouldn't try to detox at home. They aren't "good candidates" for outpatient therapy, we might say. In Andy's case, the absence of another person—a spouse, a sibling, a friend—to stay with him and watch out for signs of trouble made in-home detox particularly dicey. Now more than ever, I was aware of the importance of a support circle. To detox without one was also a tall order emotionally, apart from the physical risk. But what was the alternative? He wanted to quit; I wanted to help him. There were no other options. Zero.

"Okay, so look, I can give you a medicine that will help with the withdrawal, but you have to know this is really risky," I said.

"I know, but I gotta do something," he said.

"I agree. I want to help, but you are not the perfect candidate for doing this as an outpatient."

To say the least.

I explained my concerns: possible mental status changes, seizures, hallucinations. I told him flat out that he could die from the process.

"Well, if I keep drinking, I'm going to die, too."

Andy was probably right. Alcohol is the most widely used and misused substance in the United States. The Centers for Disease Control and Prevention attribute more than 140,000 deaths a year—more than 380 each day—to excessive alcohol use.[1] Andy was well on his way to becoming part of that grim statistic.

"I'd feel better if you weren't alone. Is there anyone that can stay with you?" I asked.

"Carol. Well, she won't stay with me. She's my ex-wife. But she can check on me."

"Like a couple times a day? Can she call you every few hours and come over if you don't answer the phone?" I said.

"Yeah. She's good like that."

It would have to do.

"So you understand the risk and still want to do it?"

"I don't have a choice."

I gave him a prescription for Librium (or chlordiazepoxide), a type of benzodiazepine. This class of drugs—"benzos"—includes better-known medications like Xanax and Klonopin. They cause sedation and are used to treat anxiety, though they carry their own risks of addiction. Librium is approved by the FDA for treatment of alcohol withdrawal. I instructed Andy to get started on a B-complex vitamin and multivitamins. And I gave him an appointment for the next afternoon.

Andy was true to his word and showed up the next day.

"How's it going?" I asked, relieved to see him.

"It sucks, but so far I'm hanging in there," he said. "How are you? Busy day?"

His question was simple and common, yet it surprised me. Here we were dealing with a life-or-death detox situation, and he was asking about me.

"Uh, thanks, yeah. I'm okay. It has been pretty busy," I said.

I talked to him about AA again, urging him to call, to seek support from others who could relate to his struggles in ways that I couldn't. I thought of my own outreach to people with MS, like Sally—how meaningful those connections had been. I wanted something similar for him.

I proceeded to administer a series of questions—the Clinical Institute Withdrawal Assessment (CIWA) Scale for Alcohol—also included in the detox article. This tool is used to gather information about common symptoms: anxiety, agitation, visual disturbance, headache, tremor, and so on. Each symptom gets a certain number of points, which are tallied up. The final score helps determine how well the patient is tolerating the withdrawal. A score that is less than eight to ten indicates minimal to mild withdrawal.

Andy's score was two. He had a slight tremor, but that was it. I couldn't believe it. I was grateful—and oh so cautious.

c⁓

The next afternoon, after another encouraging visit with Andy and another CIWA score of two, Amber showed up. I hadn't seen her in months. Kim had called, but her line was disconnected. Then she walked into the clinic without an appointment and asked to see me. Knowing her volatile situation and fearing we wouldn't be able to connect with her again, I agreed.

She had orange hair this time, ripped jeans, a cropped white T-shirt, and about a dozen bracelets that clanged together whenever she moved her hand.

"You're back," I said. "How've you been?"

"Okay, but I never got in to see the shrink," she said. "I think you're right about bipolar. I found out it runs in my family, but I got better, even without any help. I was, like, almost back to normal, and I thought maybe I didn't need medicine. I thought I could just try, like, breathing exercises or yoga or something. But now I can't sleep again." Her words ran together. If she wasn't manic yet, she was close.

"Didn't you have an appointment with the psychiatrist?"

"I don't know. Maybe . . . I think I did. I think I had some kind of appointment, but I missed it. Or I was late. I don't know, but now I'm just on some kind of waiting list. They won't give me another appointment. They said there are too many people ahead of me, not enough doctors."

I let her continue for a while. She was animated but not as irritable this time. Not as anxious.

With some effort, I determined that after her visit to the psychiatric emergency room in the fall, she had missed her follow-up appointment and been put on an indefinite waiting list for psychiatric care. She had never received treatment. She had lost her phone and failed to renew her eligibility with our clinic.

As she jumped out of her seat and demonstrated the moonwalk, slipping across the exam room floor, I considered my options. Like with Andy, they were limited. I would have to phone a friend.

Kerry answered her cell phone on the fourth ring.

Oh, thank God.

A friend since high school and now a psychiatrist in California, Kerry had helped me several times with sticky situations over the years. I told her about Amber.

"Lithium," she said. "I think it's your best bet."

"Um, really? I know it has side effects. Doesn't it have to be titrated and monitored?" I was scared. Like the detox situation with Andy, this was out of my scope of practice.

"There are other options, but it's on the four-dollar list at Walmart. It's the safest bet that's actually affordable for someone paying out-of-pocket. I can walk you through the dosing and follow-up," she said.

I agreed with Kerry's suggestion. There were no better choices. I could at least get her started, hopefully avert a full-blown manic episode, and then make some calls to see if we could get her in to see a psychiatrist. I regretted that I didn't have more psychiatric training myself. As a family doctor, I often felt I knew a little about a lot of things, but not enough about anything. During my three years of family medicine residency, after graduating from medical school, I rotated through pediatrics, internal medicine, obstetrics, gynecology, surgery, and a slew of subspecialties (rheumatology, dermatology, and orthopedics, among others). The training was diverse but not deep in any one area. After residency, I saw patients of all ages, with all manner of concerns. I usually knew my limits, knew when I needed to get help from a specialist. But so often I couldn't easily or quickly access those specialists. I was regularly jumping outside my comfort zone to treat my patients because I didn't have a choice.

Amber agreed with the plan. Lithium, fortunately, was not expensive, and it was one of the few medicines shown to be effective during mania. It could also help prevent bipolar depression and reduce the risk of suicide.

I made sure we had an updated phone number for her and provided instructions on renewing with the Medical Access Program. I wished I could spend more time understanding her living situation, her work, her friends. Was there anyone who could help her get organized—to make sure she got her medicine and took it? She needed so much more than medicine, but at least this was a start. I wrote Amber's prescription with muted optimism.

⌒

Andy came back every day as promised. Every time, his CIWA scale was two or three. Every time I saw him, I took a deep breath. Thank God.

"Have you had anything to drink?" I would ask.

"No. I wanted to, but I didn't," he would say.

"Have you called AA?" I would ask.

His answer was always the same. "No. Not yet."

We spaced out the days to two, then three. We cut back on the Librium and finally stopped it. Our visits were brief, but he was always friendly and courteous. He always asked how I was doing. I was just a little bit hopeful.

But I was worried that he didn't have enough help. I thought of my own support circle, how much I relied on so many others, especially since my diagnosis. I thought of my difficulties after the spinal tap and how I never would have managed without Don and my mom. If I had faced a substance-abuse problem, I couldn't imagine trying to get sober without a team of family and friends backing me up. At one point, Andy mentioned that he knew someone—a friend of a friend, perhaps—who was an AA sponsor, a fellow alcoholic who maintained sobriety and could provide guidance to AA newcomers as they became familiar with the program and started to work through the twelve steps. A sponsor could even give Andy long-term support.

"He said he'd help me," Andy said.

"That's great, but I still think you should try to find an AA group you can join. What you're doing . . . it isn't easy."

Andy continued to see me for maybe two months. He slipped up once and drank two beers, but he was able to get back on track. He never did get established with AA but did get some help from the sponsor.

"Andy, seriously, this is a big deal. Congratulations are in order," I said when he came in sober at the eight-week mark. He had accomplished something amazing, and he had done it without much help at all. I was impressed—and still worried.

But I rejoiced in his early success, tenuous as it might be.

CHAPTER 17

Back So Soon?

April 2010

"It's back," I told Don one morning. He was brushing his teeth, and I was pulling out a running T-shirt. "I know it was stupid to think maybe I wouldn't have this damn dizziness again, but it's back, and I hate it." I was scared, too, but it was easier to latch on to anger.

"I'm sorry," Don said in a tired voice, washing off and replacing his toothbrush in its holder. Had he done the same calculation that I had, that it had been just five months since my initial diagnosis? "At least we know what it is this time. That's something, right?"

I wasn't in a mood to look on the bright side.

"Well, sure, but could it indicate some kind of MS flare? Does this mean the meds aren't working?" I needed to share that burden of anxiety, but I also worried that I might be fueling Don's.

"It's probably stress and doesn't mean too much," Don theorized.

"Stress. Right," I said. "Well, that solves it." I sighed and unrolled a pair of socks, balancing on one foot as I put on one of the socks.

"Are you having any new symptoms?"

"Just that same awful feeling that makes every day pretty much suck," I said. "Not really anything else. A little more double vision? I don't know. But that's not new . . . and you already know I'm not sleeping well."

My lack of sleep made everything worse. Sleep is important . . . and it's not optional. Lack of adequate sleep negatively impacts mood and judgment. It definitely made me more irritable with Don and the kids, and I wondered if it contributed to my dizziness.

I had struggled with sleep on and off my entire life. Even as a child, I didn't sleep easily. I was intense and competitive, worrying about grades or an upcoming swim meet. In my three-year family medicine residency, my sleep schedule became totally dysregulated, as I tried to cope with overnight shifts every third or fourth night. I had rejoiced when I no longer had to spend nights at the hospital and, in the years since, had settled into something like a normal sleep routine—until the kids, and then MS, came along.

Chronic sleep deprivation is associated with an increased risk of mental illness, diabetes, cardiovascular disease, and even early mortality. A 2022 study showed that middle-aged and older adults should ideally get seven hours of sleep a night.[1] I aimed for seven to eight hours, but my anxiety about MS and my recurrent dizziness made it nearly impossible to get the rest I needed, even when my children didn't wake me up. Lying there, tossing and turning, sleep seemed like a beautiful room that I wasn't allowed to enter. Don, next to me, would just float right in, but I was left banging at the door.

I practiced the sleep hygiene techniques I taught my patients: go to bed and wake up at the same time every day, no caffeine in the afternoon, exercise every day. I even tried to follow the most painful rule: If you're lying in bed and can't sleep for more than fifteen to twenty minutes, get up and go to another room to do a quiet activity until you feel tired again. But even the most boring reading—the Joint National Committee's updated hypertension guidelines or an article on medical office coding practices—didn't always work.

I was jealous of my prior healthy self, oblivious to her looming demise. I saw old pictures of myself. *Look at that poor, naïve sucker. She doesn't know what's coming.* I wanted to warn her, to tell her . . .what? To enjoy every moment? To appreciate her health? To stop making plans and setting goals because she would only be disappointed? No, if I'd had the chance, I would have kept quiet, opting to let her glide along in blessed ignorance.

My fear now was not of death, but of a life stripped of joy with every moment tainted. My dizziness meant I could never forget I was sick. Even at night I couldn't escape my condition because I couldn't sleep. I didn't know if I would ever feel normal again.

I went back to see Dr. Reynard, armed with a long list of questions: Is this recurrent dizziness a flare? What does it mean is going on? Is there anything I can do? Does this mean my meds aren't working? Will these symptoms ever go away?

The resounding answers were "We don't know" and "Maybe."

He had questions for me, too. "When did the symptoms start this time?" he asked.

"I don't know exactly. Sometime last month? I mean, I've always had a little dizziness. That started when my MS started, but then it got better. Now I can't sleep, and it's worse again."

"When did it get worse?"

I hesitated, trying to pinpoint that moment, that instant when I just *knew*. I tilted my head back and looked up at the exam room ceiling, then back at Dr. Reynard.

"I can't remember when it really got bad again," I said. "Three or four weeks ago, maybe a little longer? I think it was sort of gradual. And it's not exactly dizziness. That's just the best word I can find to describe it. It's not like vertigo. It's sort of like motion sickness, but I'm not unsteady."

Dr. Reynard was typing. He had an EMR now, and the computer sat between us. He couldn't look at me anymore but had to focus on the screen, recording my answers in the electronic record. I could sympathize. I knew it was a challenge to balance eye contact with proper documentation. I resented the EMR for intruding into my visits with him and for stealing so much of my own job satisfaction at the clinic. I imagined he felt the same way.

I also reprimanded myself for being one of those patients who couldn't get her story straight or describe the symptoms in a way that was easy to document, especially in an EMR with a bunch of check boxes.

"I thought you said you got your labs done, but the last results I see were from right after your first visit here," he said, scrolling through several screens on his computer.

"I did have labs done—last week sometime," I said. I was annoyed that I couldn't get my test results. I was so accustomed to medical records getting lost, sent to the wrong place, or not sent anywhere that I had made sure to tell the lab tech exactly where to send them, circling the fax number on the lab order and even letting it slip that I was a doctor—all to no avail.

"Do you have any other symptoms?" Dr. Reynard asked.

"Well, my insomnia is worse than ever. And I had some foot numbness for a few days. It's better now—the numbness, at least," I said.

"Why didn't you call?" he asked, glancing up from the computer.

"I don't know. I didn't know if it was really a big deal or if I was just being paranoid."

I should have called. I knew it, but I had put it off. I didn't tell him that I didn't want to deal with the hassle of another MRI. I didn't want to have to change medications. I didn't tell him that I was less concerned about the MRI and even MS progression than I was about getting rid of my dizziness—getting rid of it now.

I watched Dr. Reynard click the boxes in his EMR to order the MRI. It was unavoidable.

⌒

Back in the MRI tube, I felt like I was trapped in a video game. The noises ranged from high-pitched gallops to jackhammer pounds. I imagined the MRI machine talking to me: "What's up? What's up? What's up?" Grateful for the warm blanket and the earplugs that blunted the noise, I tried to downplay expectations about my results, to maintain a neutrality that would shield me from disappointment without being too pessimistic. I took deep breaths while remaining motionless, letting my mind wander.

Thank goodness I'm not claustrophobic . . . but what if I have to sneeze or cough? What if I get the hiccups? One ill-timed yawn, and they may have to start the process all over again.

Midway through the procedure, I noticed a sharp pain in the back of my head, which was pressed against a thinly padded headrest. It felt like a massage with a barbed-wire fence. I yearned to move. I really wanted to tilt my head to one side, but I resisted the instinct to jerk my head up or squeeze the hand grip that was the only way to communicate with my captors. I tried to relax, like I do at the dentist, by remembering, *I don't have to do anything now. No patients, phone calls, e-mail messages. My only job is to lie here. How often do I get to do that?*

After the MRI was over and I was released from the tube-turned-torture-chamber, I went to change into my clothes and text Don that I would be home soon.

The radiologist, who remembered me from my last visit, welcomed me into his dark office, dimly lit from the glow of the viewing monitors.

"Back so soon?" he said.

"Unfortunately. My symptoms came back, so I did, too." I appreciated the special treatment, this opportunity to go over my MRI right after getting the test done. Usually, patients have to wait for the ordering doctor—Dr. Reynard in my case—to review the results first before they can be shared. But I had asked the radiologist, as a favor to a fellow physician, to look at the films with me in person. I was beginning to wonder if the world turned on favors.

"Let's take a look," he said.

I sat in a wheeled desk chair, and he pulled up the MRI pictures—both the new films and the older ones, for comparison—on his computer. By now I could recognize the white spots. I knew they were bad, but I needed the radiologist's guidance to recognize subtle findings, identify new versus old lesions, and point out any black holes—areas of damage beyond repair. White spots can be seen with other conditions like migraines, small strokes, and certain infections, but in my case, we knew they were from MS, given their appearance, my spinal tap results, and my symptoms.

"Here's a new one. It's small, but it definitely looks like it wasn't there last fall," he said, pointing with a pencil to a small white smudge on the film.

"That's not good," I said. "Are there others?"

"I'm not sure yet," he said, clicking through different films on his large monitor and comparing them with the pictures from my MRI in November.

"Yep. Here's another one," he said, pointing again and indicating another new white spot. "And this other one here may be new. I'm not sure."

In all, we counted at least three, maybe five new spots. *My MS is getting worse.* Each white spot indicated a new area of damage to the myelin coating my nerve cells. The MRI changes meant that already I had relapsed, and it had only been a few months. This was bad news. Very bad news.

Immediately I retreated to that place of detachment, numbness. Like the day I was diagnosed the previous November, I wanted to imagine I was hearing bad news about one of my patients. *This is Mr. Sloane we're talking about, not me. I can't be like him.*

The radiologist went on to tell me, matter-of-factly, that my medicine probably wasn't working. "I predict Dr. Reynard will want to make a change," he said. "And you know there are good meds now. It used to be that when you were diagnosed with MS fifteen years ago, you were looking at—"

Five years to a cane, ten to a wheelchair. He didn't have to finish his sentence.

"It's not that way anymore, though. And you don't even have any black holes at this point—those are much worse since they indicate permanent neurodegeneration," he said.

I was frightened of changing medicines. It didn't sound like there were good alternatives. No medicine is perfect. Effective medicines often have undesirable side effects. Still, I knew I had to take something. Research was clear that disease-modifying therapies for MS—and there were a growing number of them available—were essential to reduce the risk of getting worse. But I wasn't excited about my options. One medicine could cause liver damage, anemia, and body aches. Another increased the risk of lymphoma and leukemia. It was like that childhood game of "Would you rather?" What's worse: Freezing to death or burning? Getting mauled by hyenas or eaten by piranhas? I knew, though, that I'd *rather* take an MS medicine than allow the disease to progress. No question.

My phone rang. It was Don. I made my apologies to the radiologist for the interruption and answered.

"Hi," I said. "I can't really talk. I'm with the doctor."

"Sorry . . ."

"I've got new lesions. Gotta go."

I didn't even think about how Don would react. I had announced terrifying news with a flippancy that only fed his fear. He called again fifteen minutes later.

"Uh, are you coming? Are you coming home . . . soon?" he asked.

"Yeah, I'm just about to get in the car."

"What's—are you okay?" he asked. "Are you—can you drive?"

"Yeah, I'm dizzy but no worse than usual," I said. I heard Clara shouting in the background. "You can go deal with Clara. I'll be home soon."

When I started the car, the radio came on with Tears for Fears belting out an appropriate song, "Shout," which was exactly what I wanted to do. Those horrible white spots. This whole damn disease. I was angry, so angry. Not everyone with MS ends up like Mr. Sloane. Not everyone with MS is incapacitated and in pain. But given this early relapse, my hope for a better future was fading. MS was like a big, black cloud. You can't plan a picnic with a cloud like that. How was I supposed to live my life?

But my anger was muted by Don's reaction when I got home.

"Are you—what did they say?" he asked as I shut the door and walked into the kitchen.

Don was trying to make dinner for both kids, who were as rambunctious and demanding as ever. He held a colander, but he didn't seem to know what to do with it. He walked to hug me, still holding it, stepping over the dishes from Clara's little kitchen set, which were scattered all over the floor.

"I want a snack," she said.

"Me too," said Ella.

We ignored them.

"Well, it's the real deal, unfortunately," I said, escaping his hug after just a few seconds. I took the colander and set it in the sink.

"More lesions? Are they—" Don looked shaky, sweaty. He didn't make eye contact. Instead, he looked outside at our back porch and yard. I followed his gaze. The grass needed to be cut.

"I want a snack!" Clara demanded.

"Clara! Chill out. We're just about to have dinner," I said.

Don looked like he was having a panic attack, his hands trembling slightly. I knew he had some anxiety at baseline. He hated storms and air travel. He felt uneasy in unfamiliar settings, as I'd learned while traveling with him in India and Central America. And I could be impatient, unsympathetic. Now I felt a combination of compassion and annoyance. *Get it together! You're not allowed to be more upset than me.*

"There are other meds," I reassured him. "The radiologist says Dr. Reynard will call with a new prescription."

"I know. I'm sorry. I'm so sorry," he said, hugging me again.

"It's okay. I'll make a salad. Can you just finish the pasta? It looks like you were ready to drain it," I said, indicating the pot full of penne.

e⁓

I didn't hear from Dr. Reynard for nearly two weeks. During that time, I tried to keep so busy that I wouldn't have time or energy to analyze my plight. Patients, kids, household tasks, e-mails—I jumped from one task to the next, agitated, jittery, like I'd just gulped down six cups of coffee. Distraction was the best coping technique I could manage.

I imagined Dr. Reynard calling. Perhaps he would tell me the MRI showed some minor changes that were not unexpected and tell me to continue the medicine, which I injected into my leg or abdomen every day but tolerated without side effects. We could repeat another MRI in six months.

But most of the time, if I allowed myself a spare moment to process the MRI results, I wasn't so optimistic. I was the new NFL recruit who broke a leg during the first season. Once ambitious with great promise, now I would never be able to reach my dreams, my potential.

Back in self-preservation mode, Don tried a new rationalization. "I think there is a good chance that these so-called new white spots on the MRI are left over from the original episode last fall," he said for the fourth time, a week after the MRI.

He was trying to negotiate with himself, to keep a shred of hope alive. I got that. But there was something about his optimism— no matter how hard-won—that made me feel like crap. He was in denial—like a patient who thinks a festering foot ulcer will get better on its own. He was invalidating my experience, even though his intention was to boost my spirits. I wanted to scream at him: *Just tell me that it really, really sucks. Don't try to fix it or sugarcoat it. Just get angry along with me!*

Instead, I got angry at him. "You actually think that the new spots occurred in the time after my first MRI last fall but before I started meds? You think this all still 'counts,' somehow, as just one episode that all happened several months ago?" I said. By my tone, I might as well have added, *what is wrong with you?*

"Well, I think it's possible," he replied.

He had become my coach and cheerleader. My spontaneous husband, who normally resisted my endless efforts to plan, had developed lists of people to call when I had a flare of my symptoms and needed help. We no longer took turns getting up with Clara in the middle of the night: he always did it.

I don't know why I felt so compelled to argue, to call out his wishful thinking. Perhaps I should have let myself be swept up in his hope that this wasn't really a relapse, but I was a stickler for the truth. And I knew there was no escape.

"Come on! You're just convincing yourself of this to make yourself feel better," I said. "I have new symptoms and new MRI findings. It's a relapse. It's progression of the disease."

My argumentative streak lasted all evening. When Ella told us at dinner that she was supposed to bring a "science" book to preschool and had decided she wanted hers to be about volcanoes, Don offered to take her to Book People, a favorite local bookstore. I vetoed that idea. "Why do we have to spend more money on stuff we don't need?"

I spent the next hour making a book on volcanoes with Ella. I didn't have the energy or patience, but together we researched volcanoes on the Internet and wrote and illustrated a short paper that she dictated. A volcano—it was an appropriate symbol of our family's psychological state at the moment.

Someone named Shelly called me at work on Tuesday afternoon. She said, in a cheerful voice, that Dr. Reynard wanted to see me—I should come in the next day.

More time off work. Another waiting room.

Don drove with me back to Dr. Reynard's office the next morning. We braced ourselves for bad news.

"It's not entirely clear whether this is really a treatment failure since you've just been on the medicine for four months," Dr. Reynard told me when at last we were face-to-face. "On the other hand, you have had symptoms and MRI changes, which is disease progression in my book. And the fact that you've already seemed to relapse indicates you may have a more aggressive form of the disease."

Aggressive disease? Please don't say that. That sounds terrible. As if MS itself wasn't enough.

"So, this is definitely a relapse?" Don asked.

"Probably so. Just by choosing to do the MRI we were committing to probably changing your medication regimen if the MRI showed progression," Dr. Reynard said, looking at me.

I wanted to yell, "I told you so!" to Don, but I didn't really want to be right. I just kept thinking, *What the hell did I do to deserve this?* As if there was some sort of fairness scale out in the universe.

Dr. Reynard laid out my options:

1. A different medicine that had the side effects of possible depression, liver abnormalities, and, commonly, "flu-like symptoms."

2. A medicine that required monthly infusions, worked

beautifully, but had the slight risk of progressive multifocal leukoencephalopathy (PML), one of the weirdest of the Diseases That Really Suck—a horrible, generally fatal brain infection.

3. Continuing with my current medicine but adding monthly high-dose steroid injections.

I hated my choices. Knowing the side effects of steroids (insomnia, mood changes) and their potential long-term complications (osteoporosis, high blood pressure), I rejected that option outright. And since I knew that the risk of PML—no matter how small—would haunt me relentlessly, I opted for the medicine with the flu-like side effects.

$\sim$

"Damn, this burns. It's worse than the last medicine," I complained to Don on the first night I stabbed myself in the thigh, a couple weeks later, after completing the insurance company obstacle course and meeting with a nurse. I counted one-two-three-four as the new medicine rushed in just under my skin.

"At least it's only three times a week instead of daily injections like before," he reminded me.

At least. There's sympathy for you. I was lying in bed, propping myself up on a pillow and looking over the microscopic writing on the package insert of the new medicine. I was already aware of the long side-effect profile, but I wanted to see the section on efficacy; I needed to know this medicine would work. A chart showed that only 32 percent of people taking this medication were exacerbation-free in two years, compared to 15 percent without the medication. Basically, even if I continued these injections and tolerated having the flu all the time,

I still had a 68 percent chance of another relapse within two years. Don moved over to put an arm around me. I decided not to share this latest bit of upsetting news with him.

Instead, I questioned Dr. Reynard at my follow-up appointment. I told him about a recent tingling in my leg. It had only lasted a couple of days and gone away, but I worried it might indicate another exacerbation.

"No, probably not," Dr. Reynard said. "Transient sensory changes are usually not an indication of disease progression."

"Well, that's good, but the package insert on this new medicine says I'm really likely to relapse even if I keep up with the injections," I said.

"It's difficult to predict for any individual, but we do know that if you stay relapse-free this year, the odds get better and better that you will continue to stay relapse-free," he said. "And the most recent studies indicate that you have a 66 percent chance of staying relapse-free this year."

I liked those odds a lot better.

The package insert, like the speed-reading commentator on most pharmaceutical TV commercials, also listed a range of possible side effects: severe allergic reactions, seizures, skin damage from the injections, depression, even suicide. It was designed to appease lawyers, not to comfort patients. My doctor had chosen this medication as the best option for me. He thought it had a good chance of working and was worth the risk of the side effects. I would believe my doctor.

"There's still nothing I can do to improve my odds to avoid another relapse?" I asked.

"Just take your meds. Keep up the exercise and all your wellness activities—those are so important. We can't say why you had this new episode," he replied. "We'll get another MRI in six months. That will give us a lot more information prognostically."

So this was the new reality: injections three times a week and a lot of finger crossing. I seemed to be stuck with the dizziness. The medicine wouldn't help with it, and Dr. Reynard didn't have any suggestions for me either. The only solace I had was that when I woke up the first morning after taking the new medicine, I didn't feel like I had the flu. I felt my usual dizziness but nothing out of the ordinary. I would do my best to be grateful and not dwell on that MRI in six months.

CHAPTER 18

An Ill-Equipped Life Raft

May 2010

As I turned on my computer Monday morning, Sara Maria shared some unwelcome news. "CJ's sister called," she said. I glanced at the usual mess of papers strewn across my desk. "And . . . ?" I asked, already dreading the request.

"He was stabbed in the neck last week," she continued. "His sister said he needs pain meds and antibiotics. I've already requested his hospital records."

CJ was probably the meanest patient I had. My staff was terrified of him. A huge monster of a guy, with spikey brown hair and a booming voice, he was impatient, rude, and incredibly intimidating. He came in for various aches and pains and, ironically enough, anxiety.

"I don't give a fuck" seemed to be his favorite expression.

"I'm concerned that you missed your visit with the psychiatrist," I might say. Or "Your blood pressure is a little high today."

"I don't give a fuck," he would respond.

He was also a recovering heroin addict. I suspected he might still be abusing prescription narcotics, but he wasn't getting any from me, and he swore he was clean. I wondered why he even came into the clinic since he didn't seem interested in my advice. Maybe it was just to scare the hell out of us.

I took the hospital records from Sara Maria. "Okay," I said, trying to craft a way to get out of seeing him. I could envision the fight now: CJ shouting at me about his need for pain medicines. Me, refusing and perhaps screaming for help—"Push the security button, Sara Maria!"—as he hurled himself at me.

"Let's get the records, and let me think about this," I said. "You know, of all our patients, if we had to vote on who would be most likely to get stabbed, no doubt it would be CJ."

Sara Maria chuckled uncomfortably. We both knew that CJ was also the biggest threat to all of us.

A few minutes later, Sara Maria handed me the hospital records for CJ. They weren't helpful, which was frequently the case. In fact, we were lucky if even half the time we got any records at all. For CJ, no doctor notes were available. Most likely they had been handwritten in the hospital, and the final dictations that could someday, theoretically, make it into the electronic medical records hadn't been done yet. I found an EMS report indicating that CJ had been attacked by his neighbor, stabbed in the neck, on the right side, and had undergone emergency surgery.

"Wow, it sounds like he almost died," I said.

I then found a note from a social worker. The note was short and stated that CJ was so focused on getting more pain medication in the hospital that she couldn't complete her assessment.

"What do you want to do?" Sara Maria asked as I set down the short stack of hospital notes.

"We have to see him," I said. "I can't tell anything from these notes except that he had a serious injury. He may need pain meds or a follow-up appointment with the surgeon."

All morning we were nervous.

"Do I need to call security?" Sara Maria asked. "Should we just alert them that there could be a situation?"

"No, I think it will be okay," I said. "I'm going to keep it short and sweet, just make sure he's stable, doesn't have some kind of infection, and get labs."

We closed all the doors along the hallway and told everyone to stay in their offices. But the visit was anticlimactic, our precautions unnecessary. No roaring voice, no threats. His wound was clean and beginning to heal, and he didn't even ask for pain medicines. Because he was pale, we sent him for lab work, but he was calmer than ever, as if being stabbed had caused him to mellow out somehow. He may have even said, "Thank you," on his way out.

CJ's labs came back the next day. His hemoglobin—the molecule in red blood cells that transports oxygen from the lungs to the rest of the body and carries carbon dioxide back to the lungs—was low. For men, a normal hemoglobin level is about 13.5 to 17.5 grams per deciliter. CJ's was 6.4. He was anemic alright.

"Damn it," I said to Sara Maria when I saw the labs. "He actually looked pretty good yesterday."

He had reported feeling fairly well, and his blood pressure was normal. His heart rate had been a little fast—about ninety beats a minute—but still within normal limits. But now I was wondering if he needed a transfusion.

There isn't a clear-cut threshold for when to do a blood transfusion, but usually we would at least consider one for a hemoglobin under 7.0. At low levels of hemoglobin, vital organs, notably the heart and brain, may not get enough oxygen. And if CJ was still losing blood somehow, he could be in serious trouble.

I could have seen him back in the clinic to repeat the labs and vital signs, but I couldn't get lab results quickly, and I still didn't have the hospital records I needed to understand what had happened. He would have to go back to the ER. At least he was enrolled in the Medical Access Program provided for people with very low incomes by the city of Austin. It would cover the cost of his visit. I called him, and to my relief, he agreed to go.

Sara Maria handed me the latest ER records when I arrived at work the next day, already overwhelmed after a glance at my busy schedule. It would help our productivity numbers if everyone showed up, but it wouldn't exactly do wonders for my mental health.

CJ's records, again, were sparse. They confirmed the anemia but included no physician notes or plan. A nurse note indicated the ER doctors had considered a blood transfusion but for some reason decided against it. Best I could tell, they had verified the problem, did nothing, and sent him home. CJ, whom Sara Maria reached on the phone, verified that the ER visit had been fruitless, though he was feeling pretty well, despite the anemia. I felt like I was trying to play a complicated board game with only half the instructions. I needed more information. I needed to talk to the person who had operated on him after being stabbed.

Who was that doctor? CJ didn't know. ("You don't know his name?" "I don't give a fuck.") The ER records, of course, weren't helpful. So I launched an expedition to find and contact the surgeon. I called the medical records department at the hospital and asked them to locate and read the doctor's name off the operative report from the previous week. Once I had a name, I tried MEDLink, the hospital paging service, to connect me with the doctor. He didn't call back. I tried his office, and they told me to call MEDLink. I called MEDLink again.

Finally, the surgeon called back. He didn't understand why I was making such a fuss.

"Oh, that guy? Yeah, I talked to the ER about him yesterday. He's fine."

"He's pretty anemic," I said.

"Well, that'll get better," he said. "Why did you even check the labs?"

"I didn't know—I mean, I couldn't get records, and he looked pale. I couldn't—"

"Well, he's fine," he interrupted.

My concern seemed unwarranted. CJ had pain meds, no bleeding. We probably shouldn't have even seen him that week (and wouldn't have, except for his sister's desperate call on Monday morning). He had an appointment the following week in the surgery clinic.

I felt foolish and totally frustrated. Poor communication between health care providers is a common problem, leading to medication and treatment errors, inefficiencies, and even patient deaths. I was trying to do my part to understand what was going on with my patient, and in the end, it was counterproductive, a big waste of time.

Seeing Ana Luna, my first patient of the afternoon, did little to cheer me up. Ana was forty years old with wavy black hair, but her worn face made her look ten years older. Her red shirt had come untucked on one side from her dark pants, but she didn't seem to notice. She was there because of a fainting spell the previous week.

"I know you just talked with my medical assistant, but can you tell me what happened when you passed out?" I asked.

She hesitated. "I don't really know. I was at home, and my husband was watching TV in the next room. I just don't know. . . ."

"Do you remember what you were doing right before you fainted?"

"I was cleaning up the kitchen." She looked away, and tears formed in the corners of her eyes.

I stopped typing on my laptop and moved closer. "What is it?"

"My son . . . died," she managed, her voice catching. My eyes widened with surprise, but I stayed quiet and handed her a tissue. "That was the same day, except a month later." She stopped talking, put a hand to her face, and wiped her eyes.

I sat there with Ana Luna in silence for a moment, shaking my head slightly. "Oh, Ana, I'm so sorry. Your son—your son died a month ago from the day you fainted?"

"He was just two years old!" she sobbed, pausing again to regain some composure. "Now they want to send my daughter to jail because of the accident—and she ran away."

I was struggling to put it all together. "How old is your daughter?"

"She's seventeen. She was in the car when it was hit, but she wasn't driving. She let my son ride without a car seat, though, so now they say she's supposed to go to jail. I don't know where she is."

Time for a deep breath, I told myself, trying not to make this self-calming ritual too obvious.

"Oh, Ana, I'm so sorry." I thought of my children. A daughter implicated in the death of her sibling. But I couldn't go there, not really. I had to summon that professional distance. It was something that came up in medical school, the idea of respectful boundaries. Don't get involved. Don't share personal information. For heaven's sake, don't give out your cell phone number.

But I was still human. I could allow a little bit of empathy to seep in—it would help me connect with her, allow her to feel understood. We spend our lives building a sandcastle—piling on the sand, shaping the walls, the roof, the towers. We know that the tide will eventually come in and wash it away, but we still enjoy the process of sculpting and making it beautiful. In her case, someone had stepped on her castle far too soon. I could share her sadness, her devastation. Nevertheless, I had to limit its influence. And I had to be able to turn it off later, to let it go.

"I don't know—I don't know where she is!" she said again, crying softly.

"Okay, okay. That must be so scary. I'm sure she's scared, too, but I bet she'll come back soon." I paused, blinking away tears from my own eyes. "Do you have other children?"

She nodded. "Two more. My other daughter's nine, and I have a son who's almost fifteen."

"Okay, and I imagine this is hard on them, too. But you know what? You need to be able to take care of them, and you can't do that if you don't take care of yourself. Let's start your exam."

I went through the motions of a heart and lung exam, also including a detailed neurologic exam for good measure. Everything was normal. I often saw patients with physical symptoms—abdominal pain, headaches, generalized pain—that could only be explained by mental health disorders, like depression and anxiety. Often I struggled to sort out what was a result of a physical illness versus a psychiatric condition. But in this case, I felt confident that Ana Luna's grief and worry, rather than a brain tumor, stroke, or heart arrhythmia, had caused her to faint.

I grappled with the decision to start her on an antidepressant. She was clearly miserable, but many doctors would consider her to have an "adjustment disorder"—an emotional or behavioral reaction to a stressful life event or change. With such a clear trigger for her symptoms, major depression, which comes on more gradually and lasts longer, seemed less likely, though the lines between the two conditions were blurry, and overlap was possible.

I thought of those terms. Neither was adequate. Adjustment disorder. How do you adjust to the death of a child? Her reaction seemed perfectly appropriate, not some kind of disorder. And major depression. This was certainly "major," but it went far beyond depression. She was living in hell, and Prozac probably wouldn't do much. Ultimately I ordered labs, asked Sara Maria to do an electrocardiogram to help rule out an arrhythmia, and referred her to our part-time counselor, a new and much-welcome addition to our team. We scheduled a follow-up appointment for the next week without starting any medicine.

The rest of the afternoon went as smoothly as could be expected. But during my second-to-last patient visit, as I was discussing the significance of a young woman's menstrual irregularities and abnormal hormone levels, Don called. I normally wouldn't have answered in the middle of a patient encounter, but I excused myself from the room and got the news I'd dreaded.

"The vet says it's time to say goodbye to Mocha," Don said, his voice breaking. Don had taken our twelve-year-old dog to the vet that afternoon after she'd collapsed the previous night. Mocha, who we adopted from the Houston animal shelter when we were in medical school, before we were married, had been our first kid. She had followed us to the three different apartments and two different houses we'd lived in over the years, and until just a few years ago, she had been my most reliable running companion.

I could not let myself process what Don was saying. "I'll call you right back. I have to finish seeing this patient."

I went back in the room and concluded the visit as quickly as possible. Then I called Don back. "What did they say?" I asked, still unwilling to let myself be sad.

"The vet noticed that Mocha's abdomen was distended. She stuck a needle in—it was full of blood. Then they did an x-ray. Mocha has cancer all over her lungs."

"Can I come see her?" I held back tears. "I've just got one more patient."

"Yeah, they can keep her here for a while."

I hung up and rushed into the last exam room.

Carlos was sitting on the exam table. He was a wreck—disheveled and sweaty. He looked like I felt.

"Hey, what's going on? How are you doing?" I asked, settling on my stool.

"Terrible," he said. "I'm getting kicked out of my house, I'm out of my medicines, and I feel like shit. They turned me down for disability again."

"Okay, that's a lot. I'm sorry to hear it," I said. "What medicines are you out of?"

"All the psych meds. I ran out three days ago, and I'm having panic attacks again," he said, his voice rushed and anxious.

I glanced at his med list, but I struggled to concentrate. *I've got to get out of here. He's a mess, but so am I. I need to get to Don and see my dog. My sweet dog.*

I took a breath. I had to rein myself back in. *Save the meltdown for later. Don't go there now.*

"Carlos, your meds are all generics. You can get them at Walmart for four dollars each."

"Yeah, but I have one dollar and fifty-four cents. My sister's kicking me out. My family is useless. They won't lend me money. My dad told me yesterday that he wishes I would die, and he never wanted me anyway."

"Oh man, that sucks!" I replied. *Really,* I told myself, *as bad as I feel, as rushed as I am to get to the vet, I need to listen to what this guy is saying. He deserves my attention and compassion.* I took another deep breath and forced myself to focus on at least the one problem for Carlos that I could fix.

"It's pretty clear to me that you're having withdrawal from the psych meds, especially the Celexa," I said. "It's called discontinuation syndrome. It happens a lot if you stop the medicine too suddenly. Let me see what I can do."

I was angry but not at Carlos. Maybe it was his fault. Maybe he didn't make the best decisions, but did that really matter? It certainly wouldn't help to punish him by depriving him of important medicine. Elected officials love to brag that the U.S. health care system is "the best in the world." Yet my clinic, in some ways, had more in common with the clinics where I'd worked in Honduras and India during my medical training than private practices in the affluent West Lake Hills neighborhoods across town. These same officials also complained loudly at any suggestion of rationing health care as a cost-saving measure. Yet at that very moment, people were paying big bucks for Botox in West Lake while Carlos couldn't pay four dollars for his anxiety medicine.

Carlos deserved some credit for seeking treatment for his anxiety in the first place. According to the American Psychiatric Association, less than half of the people who need it obtain mental health care. Men are notoriously resistant to getting help. Due to innumerable barriers, including stigma, lack of insurance, and a shortage of racially diverse and culturally competent providers, people of color, like Carlos, are even less likely to get the care they need. In a 2008–2015 survey, only 31 percent of Blacks and Hispanics with mental illness received services compared to 48 percent of whites.[1]

He had overcome so much to get help in the first place. We couldn't desert him now.

I left Carlos in the exam room to go brainstorm solutions with Sara Maria. Were there any samples of Lexapro (similar to Celexa) that would be a reasonable substitute? No. Could we get medicines through the community clinic pharmacy for free, and they could bill him later? No. Was there a social worker we could contact for emergency assistance with medical costs and housing? No, as our chain of community clinics didn't have a social worker. Did anyone have three dollars so Carlos could at least get one of the meds, the Celexa, at Walmart? Yes. That we could do. A quick office collection ensued. Flashes of advice from prior colleagues and instructors came to me: "Don't get too involved. Keep your distance. Don't become friends with patients." I didn't think they would approve of the gift of three dollars to Carlos, but then again, my dog was dying, and my patient was facing homelessness.

"Really?" Carlos said as I handed him the money.

"I haven't done this before and probably won't do it again," I said, "But you need your medicines now more than ever." I paused. "You know, you're a smart guy. You're young, too. You're not terribly disabled—you just can't do physical labor anymore because of your lung problems. But you could do something else."

"I love music—I'd love to teach music," he confessed.

"Yeah? You could get a degree at the community college and teach music."

"No one's ever told me I'm smart before," he said.

"You have the potential to do a lot. You don't need disability. . . ." My voice trailed off.

"Music—I'd be happy teaching music." He was visibly calmer.

"Yeah, that'd be really cool," I said. It was unrealistic, sure, but as I had learned in my own battles with dizziness and despair, just the hope of achieving a goal can be motivating. "Get your meds now, get your housing situation worked out, and then look into that option," I continued. "Carlos, let me see you back in two months. I'm hoping things will settle down for you by that point."

I darted back to my desk, turned off my computer, and jotted down a reminder to finish the note from Carlos's visit later. Then I headed to the veterinary clinic.

I rushed inside and was ushered back to the room where Don sat next to Mocha, looking sadder than I'd ever seen him. I hugged him—a long, clinging hug. Then I turned to Mocha, who lay nearly motionless on the floor. I sat next to her and stroked her back, crying quietly as the vet injected our sweet dog with a life-ending drug. Remembering the day we'd first found her at the Houston animal shelter, a scared little thing—all legs, tail, and funny, floppy ears—Don and I now watched her die.

⌒

By Friday, Sara Maria, Terri, and I were exhausted. Kim had been out all week, and our other new medical assistant had been pulled out at the last minute for extra training off-site. We were all behind, and we stayed late, working into the evening.

The new productivity numbers were in, and we were no closer to our goal. Would our affiliated community clinics want to back out of our partnership? Would I be able to keep my job? I dreaded the conversation with the administration but planned my defense. I would tell them we needed more nurse time and major improvements to the EMR. I would tell them that Ana Luna and Carlos and even CJ deserved more than ten or fifteen minutes of face time with me when coming in for a visit. I would explain that short visits and quality care were incompatible; to expect both was like expecting fine dining at a fast-food restaurant. As much as I hated to be behind schedule, I would rather run late than lower my standards and provide subpar care. But I didn't expect a sympathetic response.

A former colleague once told me about his international elective in Kenya during medical school. The doctor with whom he was working—the only doctor at the hospital—left him in charge during a multiday trip to get supplies in Tanzania. When a patient came in with a gangrenous arm, my colleague, still just a student, had made a decision to amputate. I had been horrified at the thought of it.

"But you had no idea what you were doing. You weren't trained in surgery!" I had exclaimed.

"I got a book. I got a nurse to help. The patient would have died without the operation. There was no one else. I did what I had to do," he'd answered.

That was it—there was no one else. I had gotten this job—directing a clinic for people without private insurance—because no one else wanted it. I felt like an ill-equipped life raft, rushing from one sinking ship to the next. I regretted my lack of training, my lack of mentors, to prepare me to be that life raft. But even though I felt like damaged goods—afflicted by chronic dizziness and increasing white spots, with the specter of MS black holes planted on my shoulders—I

CHAPTER 19:

Sprouts and Eggs

July 2010

A ll summer, as I sat in traffic, ran at the lake, or struggled to sleep, I couldn't stop asking the ultimate question, the one that plagues many of us with serious medical problems: *Why me? Why did I get MS?*

"You're the healthiest person I know," a fellow mom from Ella's preschool class had told me when she heard about my diagnosis. "I mean, you're a vegetarian, you run every day, you don't even drink."

She didn't know about my weakness for French fries from Hyde Park Bar and Grill and for Upper Crust cinnamon rolls, but I did prioritize my health—I'd give her that.

"Life isn't fair," I would tell Ella and Clara when they complained about a perceived injustice: an early bedtime, an uneven distribution of snacks. But somehow I still felt angry, wronged by my diagnosis. This dizziness—this whole dreadful disease—seemed to have pushed

201

my life onto an entirely different path than I'd planned. I'd had a good plan, and I'd worked hard to make it happen. MS wasn't part of the plan.

I did have a couple strikes against me. MS is two to three times more common in women, and while it can occur at any age, most often it affects people twenty to fifty years old. Epstein-Barr virus (EBV), the cause of infectious mononucleosis (mono), was being investigated as a potential trigger for MS, with mounting evidence of a link. I wondered if having mono in high school could have caused MS to develop nearly twenty years later.

But I lacked other risk factors: smoking, family history, other autoimmune disease, living in the northern part of the country. Surely, I wasn't always destined to have MS. Even if EBV could trigger MS, why did it happen to me? Most people who get EBV are fine. So what was the inciting event, the very first thing that caused my immune system to attack my central nervous system? Was it because I was a vegetarian, as the acupuncturist had implied some months earlier? Was it from some toxic exposure during our home remodel or some other environmental pollutant? Had I become vitamin D deficient by spending so much of my young adulthood indoors, training to be a doctor? Was it from stress, sleep deprivation, soy, or gluten? Maybe I picked up a parasite on a trip to the Amazon during residency. Maybe I got some weird infection from accidentally eating spoiled food. Or could it even be from not drinking alcohol? Was I too much of a Goodie-Two-shoes?

Much of my speculation was not at all scientifically based. It didn't even make sense. But traditional medicine had failed me. It couldn't provide an explanation or a cure. I never missed a dose of my medication, and still I had relapsed. My prescriptions didn't help my dizziness, and even the more mainstream alternative therapies, like acupuncture and yoga, offered only short-term relief.

My relapse had proved that I couldn't stop further MS progression. Uncertainty was a big part of my life now, and I was adjusting to that reality by trying to be more flexible, less tied to a preferred outcome. There seemed to be something akin to grace in this understanding, especially when I eventually allowed myself to stop asking *Why me?* It would serve me well later, especially during the COVID pandemic, when we all faced a level of insecurity we had never expected. But even as I began to accept a higher degree of uncertainty, I was relentless in search of a remedy for the persistent, miserable dizziness that continued to haunt me most days, interfering with my work, my mood, my relationships.

I expected it now. Even when I woke up feeling normal, the dizziness would creep back by midmorning and surround me with a dim cloud, a constant buzz that made everything more exhausting and overwhelming.

I was thinking all sorts of crazy things, like how I might prefer a more obvious disability. With a cane, a sling, or a brace, maybe I'd garner sympathy. I didn't want sympathy, not exactly—and I certainly didn't want a physical disability. I know how awful that sounds just to mention it. What I craved, though, was understanding—from the clinic administrator who called my cell phone when I was two minutes late to a meeting, from the kids when I asked for help cleaning up their toys and clothes strewn all over the house, from Don when I needed a break from meal preparation or running errands. My dizziness was invisible and impossible to explain. No one wanted to hear about it. And because most days I was capable of *acting as if*—I could fake my way through meetings, patient care, and family activities—I didn't give myself a break either. Every day was worse because of that damn dizziness. On the rare days when I didn't feel dizzy, the threat of it hovered nearby, sapping my motivation. I didn't know which was worse.

I became the subject of my own research experiment. Tracking my symptoms on a scale of one to ten, I would rate how I felt each day, looking for correlations with sleep and stress. I wanted to uncover the mystery of why I would be so affected on some days and not others. Was I feeling off-kilter because I hadn't slept well? Maybe. But what about the days when, after being up much of the night because of Clara or just insomnia, I would be fine? Surely I could find the magic potion to keep it at bay.

Encouraged by a doctor friend with an interest in alternative medicine, I decided to try an elimination diet. By that point, I had read enough to know that many in the MS community were enthusiastic about a whole slew of anti-inflammatory and other creative diets, which were credited with miracle cures, triumphant recoveries. According to some dietary gurus, gluten, breakfast cereal, and white rice were out; avocados, ginger, and walnuts possessed properties that would reduce inflammation and could prevent MS relapses. I was skeptical but desperate.

Like the name implies, the elimination diet is a highly restricted diet that seeks to identify problematic food by cutting out anything that could conceivably cause an allergy, a digestive problem, or other symptoms. Initially, almost everything is off-limits. Then, after a few weeks, different foods are gradually added back into the diet, while monitoring for symptoms. While I still struggled to see the connection between dizziness and wheat or cheese, for example, I also recalled what I sometimes said to patients about diet: If one or two little pills a day can control your diabetes or prevent a heart attack, imagine the great impact that healthier food might have. On the off chance that the elimination diet would help, I gave it a try.

I ate nuts, fruits, and vegetables for a month. I was already a vegetarian, but now I stopped dairy, gluten, sugar, and caffeine as well.

"Why are you doing this again?" Don asked when I refused another request to go out to dinner because I knew I wouldn't be able to find an acceptable meal.

"Apparently, a lot of people find that cutting out certain foods helps reduce annoying symptoms. And you know, there are all those MS diets out there that are supposed to prevent progression. Maybe this makes a little bit of sense, and I can come up with my own MS diet," I said.

I was sorry to inconvenience Don, but I was also irritated with the implication that my idea was crazy. It wasn't as if he had come up with a better plan. I was sensitive to his judgment because I thought the elimination diet was a little wacky myself. I also thought that while I might be inconveniencing him, he should just suck it up because MS was inconveniencing me a lot more.

I sought out gluten-free, sugar-free granola. I stocked up on coconut milk yogurt because my usual Greek yogurt was forbidden. I read nutrition labels, bought massive amounts of organic produce, and found recipes involving quinoa, kale, and other permissible food. When I relented to go out for a family brunch, I ordered a side dish of fruit, longing for a sip of my sister's cappuccino. Thanks to my inner drill sergeant, I resisted the temptation.

The first week I felt a little better. Was it helping? No. The second week was worse. Maybe I still needed more time. Maybe I was "detoxifying" and would feel better in a few more days. But at the end of four weeks, my dizziness showed no pattern or indication of improvement; like my MS, it was out of my control. I couldn't add different foods back in to see if they caused a return of symptoms because the symptoms had never gone away in the first place. Maybe for some people serious dietary changes and restrictions do relieve symptoms and reduce disease progression. I didn't want to discount their experiences. But for many, I thought, the "success" of various MS diets was because of the natural course of relapsing, *remitting* MS. Although neurologic damage may accumulate over time, the progression is more wavelike than linear.

When I reintroduced gluten and dairy back into my diet, I felt exactly the same. I still found reason to celebrate, however. The elimination diet was awful. I went back to Central Market to stock up: Greek yogurt, buns for veggie burgers, whole-wheat tortillas, all the ingredients for homemade granola. I was delighted to eat regular food again.

Discouraged, but undeterred, I decided to keep searching. Something *had* to make my symptoms better. My next strategy was to try a special kind of physical therapy for people with dizziness and balance problems. Another doctor friend had suggested it, telling me the story of a woman whose crippling vertigo had been cured by balance therapy involving ballroom dancing. It sounded strange but worth a try.

The physical therapist was a tall woman in her late fifties. She had short gray hair, no makeup, and was a bit awkward, as if she hadn't been doing this long, though I knew she had.

"I wanted to see if you could help me with my dizziness," I told her. "It seems weird that physical therapy might help, but I am willing to try almost anything."

I sat with the therapist in a standard exam room, reviewing my history, and she seemed to gain confidence and authority as we went along. She asked all the basic questions about how long I'd had dizziness, what it felt like, and what made it worse.

"It's better when I'm running, oddly enough," I said. "But if I'm stretching afterwards and lean over, it seems worse. Looking up also makes it a little worse."

She jotted down some notes and then launched into a thorough neurologic exam, concluding with a test that was unfamiliar to me. She told me to read a line of letters off the usual eye chart with the big E at the top. No problem. Then she held my head in both hands and moved it from side to side quickly.

"Now, read the lowest line you can," she instructed.

I couldn't focus on the eye chart. The letters were moving all over the place. I could sort of make out the third lowest line, and with much hesitation I read the letters. This seemed like a normal result to me, and I was surprised when she told me it was not.

"I think you're having problems with your vestibulo-ocular reflex," she said. "This would explain most of what you've described and explain your test results, except I'm not sure how to account for the fact that you feel better when you're running. Usually that would make things worse."

Vestibulo-what? I didn't know what the vestibulo-ocular reflex was, but I gathered that it had something to do with balance and vision, so I played along. She continued with another head-shaking exercise and more tests. Then the computer generated some graphs of my results that looked like Clara's scribbles.

Glancing at the squiggly graphs, the physical therapist nodded, as if the tests confirmed her earlier suspicions. I didn't know what to think. *Is this real medicine?*

The therapist launched into a lengthy discussion of my vestibulo-ocular reflex, which, I learned, was supposed to stabilize images when I moved my head. She named various tests and therapies I might try. I thought of my patients' blank stares sometimes when I tried to explain medical concepts that I thought were easy and obvious. I almost wished the therapist hadn't known that I was a doctor so she would have simplified her explanation. "I know I'm supposed to understand this, but right now I'm at about a third-grade level," I wanted to say. Instead, I, like many of my patients, feigned understanding, embarrassed to share the extent of my ignorance.

The therapist taught me some exercises: stare at the letter *K* in the middle of a page of letters. Shake your head back and forth for fifteen seconds. Stop, then repeat the whole thing two more times, a little faster each time. Then repeat the process while nodding your head up and down.

It was weird, but if she had told me to go skydiving or switch to a diet of only sprouts and eggs to stop my dizziness, I probably would have done it. I could understand the success of businesses promising sensational cures for a myriad of ailments through herbs, supplements, magnets, or crystals. Traditional medicine can be frustratingly limited.

As with the elimination diet, I followed the recommendations for my physical therapy with an obsessive commitment. My vestibulo-ocular reflex would be forced to comply; I would whip it into shape. To do my exercises, I would stand on a pillow or couch cushion and stare at letters on a piece of paper while shaking my head, first back and forth, then up and down. Don and the kids would laugh at me until I banished them from the room.

The more effort we put into a project, the more likely we are to believe we are successful. We value the sourdough bread we've made from scratch more than the store-bought variety, the handmade Valentine's Day card more than the one from Hallmark. A high-priced, six-step skin-care regimen is bound to yield better perceived results than a cheap bar of soap, simply because it's expensive and time-consuming. We want to believe our extra work is worth something, so we do. But even with great effort, I finally had to concede the balance exercises—my vestibulo-ocular reflex training program—were a failure. As Dr. Reynard told me when we discussed it, I was going to have to learn to live with the dizziness. He didn't say it, but I knew I should be glad my symptoms weren't any worse.

CHAPTER 20:

I Didn't See It Coming

August 2010

One of my patients was a murderer. Sara Maria saw the story on a local news station one evening in late July and told me the next day at the clinic.

"I mean, Marcus? He's, like, one of my nicest patients," I said. Sara Maria couldn't believe it either.

I googled the news story. Apparently Marcus and his son were involved in an altercation with a security guard, during which Marcus had allegedly smashed the guard over the head with a concrete block. Alcohol may have been involved.

I was dumbstruck and distressed. He had been upbeat and friendly at his last appointment just a couple months earlier. I remembered our visit because I'd been impressed that Marcus had made a real effort to improve his health. He had brought in a blood pressure log to review—a calendar with readings from almost every day, showing

UP the DOWN Escalator

excellent control of his hypertension. With pride, he shared that he was exercising daily, had reduced his salt intake, and was eating better.

I wondered if I could have seen it coming. Did I advise him about alcohol? Could I have counseled him about anger management? Was I really such a poor judge of character?

But maybe it wasn't my oversight at all. Maybe it was the perfect, awful combination of poverty, hopelessness, and fear that pushed him over the edge.

I thought of him in prison. Terror. Guilt. And what about his wife? Had I met her? Perhaps at Marcus's first visit? I thought of calling her, but what would I have said?

Of course, another family had lost someone, too, under the worst possible circumstances. A whole invisible line of relatives, friends, coworkers—the people behind the headline—were out there somewhere, shocked, grieving. They didn't see this coming . . . and then it happened. So wrong, permanent. No way to prepare. No way to take it back. Like so many things that impact our lives, in big ways and small ones. Like getting MS—and not at all like that.

And I couldn't dwell on it any longer because a new administrator, the latest in a long string of people assigned to us as our "practice manager," had arrived to talk to Kim and me about the upcoming audit.

The audit was a big deal. The Joint Commission on Accreditation of Healthcare Organizations was coming to evaluate us in two weeks. My clinic and all our affiliated community clinics were likely to be visited, and no fire extinguisher should be unchecked or electrical outlet left uncovered. If the hand sanitizer was expired, we'd get big black marks. If a staff member incorrectly stated, to the all-knowing inspector, which part of the parking lot was designated as a safe zone during an evacuation, we were doomed. We were like panicked airline passengers who had just been told to prepare for a crash landing.

I was annoyed. Really annoyed, all the more so because I knew the stress, and especially my anger at the administrators and the process, were not good for my health. I didn't need the Joint Commission to provoke an MS exacerbation.

A few weeks before, someone from the administration had marched in and removed all the medications we kept on hand for emergencies. We could keep the aspirin, but they took the lisinopril and hydrochlorothiazide—medicines that I might dispense if a patient showed up with high blood pressure after forgetting or running out of her usual medicine. The small stash of antibiotics, for treating bladder infections and pneumonia, was removed.

"These medicines aren't on the 'approved list,'" he'd said, confiscating everything.

Someone else had removed the tiny vials from the exam rooms that we needed to do pap smears, proclaiming them a "hazard." We weren't even allowed to have the one-inch individually packed alcohol swabs in the rooms unless they were locked up. "If a child put that in her mouth, it could be dangerous," we were told. The colorful wooden mobile that I had hung from the ceiling of our new pediatric exam room was removed out of a concern that it could fall on someone. Our donated used children's books that we distributed to the kids who came in the clinic? They were a menace. Each book had to be washed by a volunteer and kept in a basket in the front office to be handed one-by-one to select families. The kids could no longer look through the books and select their favorites.

It was a caution taken to the most ridiculous extreme. And there was more.

At a monthly meeting of the community clinics, the medical director told all the doctors and nurse practitioners that the Joint Commission required us to introduce ourselves to patients when we entered an exam room. *Reasonable enough*, I thought. But he went on to explain that we were required to ask each patient for two "identifiers" (full name and date of birth, for example) at every visit. Okay, I could see the point of doing this for new patients or those undergoing medical procedures. But we were supposed to do this for all patients at all visits even if we had just seen them the previous day and a hundred times before that. Even if I knew the intricate details of someone's life, including her recent extramarital affair and that funny-looking mole on her inner thigh, I was supposed to introduce myself like we'd never met and ask for her full name and date of birth. If I didn't, it would be another big black mark. Those who refused to comply, the medical director said, should consider working elsewhere.

The Joint Commission was important—I got that. They were there to protect patients from medical mishaps. I certainly wouldn't want to end up with the wrong prescription or someone else's lab results when I went to see Dr. Reynard. And it may very well have been the administration's interpretation of the rulebook that was ridiculous rather than the rules themselves.

But the whole time we were planning for their arrival, I couldn't stop thinking that the Joint Commission, and the administrators that were overseeing our preparation, were missing the point. I felt like my team and I were racing through a blizzard to take someone to the emergency room, yet we risked getting pulled over for having a crooked license plate.

When Don and I were in medical school, he was assigned to two different physicians in small towns near Houston to complete his family medicine rotation. The first doctor, we later found out, was under order from the Texas Medical Board to never be alone in a room with a patient because he had assaulted too many of them. Years later, he was convicted of insurance fraud for setting fire to his house, car, and eventually his medical practice. Shouldn't our quality-control efforts be focused on people like that rather than children's books and unnecessary identity checks?

Then there was Don's other family medicine instructor. One day during Don's two weeks with him, the doctor himself had fallen ill. He had developed a concerning heart rhythm and was admitted to the hospital for further testing. Instead of canceling his patient appointments for the day, he summoned Don to his hospital bed where he handed him a pre-signed prescription pad. "Here you go. Thanks," he'd said. Don—a third-year medical student—was left alone in the office to see all the patients.

Presumably, these weren't isolated incidents. Yet there we were, obsessively removing test kits from our exam rooms because of some perceived threat and memorizing inane rules that would do nothing to help our patients. I almost wanted to quit.

᠃

I barely had time to acknowledge my own birthday in early August as I rushed that morning to get Clara to preschool and Ella to summer dance camp. Packing lunches, Joint Commission, Marcus, possible dizziness cures . . . all were competing for my attention.

Cathy called to sing "Happy Birthday" over the phone as I finished dropping off Ella at Dance Discovery and started the drive to Clara's preschool. Then, while I was settling Clara in her classroom, I answered a call from Sara Maria.

"Lisa, we've got a situation here." Sara Maria's voice sounded some-what amused over my cell phone.

"I'll be there in ten minutes, but what's the situation?" I asked.

"We have Mike here."

"What?" I couldn't hear her well, surrounded by the shrieks of two-year-olds and Clara's tugs on my sleeve. "Just a second, Clara," I whispered. "Sorry, Sara Maria. You said Mike? Forget it, I'll be right there."

On the way to the clinic, I tried to figure out what Sara Maria was talking about. Who was Mike? She had sounded cheerful, so it wasn't anything bad. Maybe she had a birthday breakfast planned and wanted me to hurry up?

Sara Maria had left beautiful, fragrant lilies on my desk, but she was not in surprise-party mode, I soon discovered.

"So what were you talking about—Mike who?" I asked, tossing my workbag under my desk.

"No. Not 'Mike.' *Mice.* We have mice here," she said.

"The mouse was so cute," Lina, our new medical assistant, chimed in. "It's been running around the exam rooms."

I sighed. "I don't think the Joint Commission will think it's cute."

Sara Maria had already called Building Services. They would be sending a rodent exterminator to catch the mice and decontaminate the rooms.

"We're not supposed to use those exam rooms where the mouse was," Lina said.

"So the admin team knows about this, too?" I asked.

"Yes, and they aren't happy," Sara Maria replied.

"Can you even imagine the trouble we'd be in if the Joint

Commission spotted a mouse in here?" I asked, smiling. "I think they'd probably pull out handcuffs and arrest us all."

"Really," Sara Maria said, chuckling.

⌒

The mice were long forgotten by the time the Joint Commission arrived in Austin the following week. I started getting texts early in the morning—every move made by the Joint Commission auditors was tracked and reported widely, as if they were the president and his entourage. "They went to see Magnolia Clinic. We expect they may come to you next," one text read. Then, "Make sure the sharps containers are hung properly in the exam rooms and aren't overfilled." Then, "They're off to Eastern Hills."

For three days, I imagined blaring trumpets announcing their arrival at the clinic as self-assured, well-groomed men accompanied by bodyguards in suits and sunglasses glided into the lobby. Being the daughter of a congressman, I knew how to greet important visitors. A smile, eye contact, and a firm handshake were needed when meeting presidential candidates and U.S. senators. I knew to project confidence, speak clearly, add a little humor—but not too much. I planned to race up to the front to welcome the Joint Commission, acting like I could barely contain my delight. I would lead them through the clinic as they admired the newly polished floors and friendly staff. They would check the cabinets and say, "Ah, you even locked up the alcohol swabs." And I would smile and say, "Yes, of course. It would be far too dangerous to keep accessible alcohol swabs in an exam room. A child might poison herself."

But they never came. I think I was the only one who was

disappointed that of the twenty-some community clinics, ours was one of two that wasn't visited.

c⁓

I was startled to see Marcus's name on my schedule a few days later. I had thought he was in prison, but he showed up for the appointment.

"His blood pressure's up," Sara Maria said, handing me the intake form.

"So do you think he's out on bail?" I asked.

"I guess," Sara Maria replied. "He didn't say anything to me."

With the Joint Commission still in mind, I apologetically asked for two identifiers, after my initial greeting. He rattled off his name and birthday. He didn't have his blood pressure log. He had run out of one of his medicines. He said he felt fine and denied any new concerns. Was I imagining his aura of apathy?

Marcus didn't mention the murder accusation, and I wasn't about to bring it up. I cleaned my stethoscope with an alcohol swab from my pocket and went through the motions of listening to his heart and lungs. Feeling just a little uneasy, I refilled his blood pressure medicine. *Does he know that I know?* He was polite as always, but I sensed a distance and tension that hadn't been there before.

I wasn't there to judge. I didn't know the story. To hell with the Joint Commission's silly rules that had shifted my focus to expiration dates on hand sanitizer and approved cleaning products. My job was to listen to as much or little as he wanted to share and to provide the best care I could. But when I bid Marcus goodbye, I think I knew I would never see him again.

CHAPTER 21:

Your Call Is
Important to Us

October 2010

"Thank you for calling. We apologize for the delay. Your call is important to us. Please remain on the line, and your call will be answered in the order it was received."

My MS medicine was late. It should have arrived the day before, in a big cardboard box with my name on it. I was glad I still had a week's supply at home in my refrigerator, but I didn't understand the delayed delivery.

Most MS medicines are specialized medicines that are only available at specialized mail-order pharmacies and cost about the same as a midrange used car for a three-month supply. Fortunately, I had an insurance company that covered most of the cost, and the specialized pharmacy usually got the medicine to me on time, packed in a large Styrofoam cooler, as if they were delivering a new heart or kidney.

Now, after navigating a phone tree that felt like a corn maze, I was waiting for a live human to pick up the phone.

"All available representatives are assisting other customers. Please stay on the line for the next available agent," the cheerful recorded voice said on the other end of the line.

"Of course they are. And I can tell my call is very important to you. After all, I've only been waiting for sixteen minutes," I said into the receiver.

Then I heard the music again. The music, computer-generated with forced jollity, was grating, barely more pleasant than Ella's whines when I tried to get her to practice the piano.

"Thank you for calling Enjoy Your Wait Pharmacy. How may I assist you?" another cheerful voice—this time a real one—said on the other end of the line.

"Yes, hi. I was calling to clarify why my medication didn't get delivered yesterday," I said, faking cheerfulness as well.

"I should be able to help you with that. May I get your name and member ID?"

I gave her both.

"Thank you. Please be patient for one moment while I look you up in our system."

I waited. At least she didn't put the hold music back on.

"I apologize, but I am not finding that member ID in our system," she said after a minute or so.

"Well, I have it right here in front of me." I repeated the number, and she confirmed that was what she tried. I imagined my patients trying to get refills, schedule radiology tests, pay hospital bills. Navigating the phone tree was hard enough for me, and I spoke English and had postgraduate degrees. I was a doctor, and it was still exasperating!

"Let's try looking you up with your date of birth," she suggested.

Why didn't we just do that in the first place?

I gave her my date of birth, waited another minute, and felt genuinely cheerful when she said, "Here you are! Lisa Doggett. And oh yes, your member ID is here, too. You're not supposed to include the 'T' in front of it."

Then why did they print a T in front of the number on my card? Oh, it must be a silent T, like the K in the word "know." I should have "Known." But we were getting somewhere, and I kept my mouth shut.

"So which medication were you calling about?" she asked.

"I only have one—for my MS. It was supposed to be delivered yesterday."

"Okay, yes. For that medicine, you will need to speak with Phone Trees R Us Pharmacy. They are the ones who handle deliveries for the specialized medications. I'd be happy to give you that phone number," she said.

My frustration building, I dialed the new number. Perhaps I should have known which pharmacy to call. I had called the pharmacy number on my insurance card first, not giving it much thought. But I was learning now from personal experience what my patients—at least those with insurance—had been telling me for years: dealing with insurance companies was not intuitive, efficient, patient centered, or friendly.

"Thank you for calling Phone Trees R Us Pharmacy. Please note that our menu options have changed. Please listen to the following options before making your selection."

Here we go again!

The new phone tree was like a Choose Your Own Adventure book. Did I want to listen to the message in English or Spanish? Was I calling about a new prescription or a prescription refill? Did I want to make a payment, arrange for a shipment of medication, update my contact information, or speak with a nurse or pharmacist?

I clicked the "8" on my phone to "check the status of an order." Did I want to update my shipping address, update my payment address, update my insurance information, or report a problem with my order? *A problem with my order . . . yes!* I clicked the "4" and was promptly disconnected.

With a deep breath, I called back, furious, but trying to remain calm. When the phone tree started again, I refused to climb. I just kept pushing the "0" hoping to get an operator. Instead, I kept getting re-routed back to the same menu. I felt like I was trapped in a sticky web.

I had to listen to the phone tree options again, ultimately selecting "speak to a pharmacist." At least I could hopefully get a person on the line.

"We are experiencing an unusually high call volume. Please remain on the line and the next available pharmacy staff person will assist you."

About once a month I actually took a lunch break. This was my break. I pounded my head on the desk. At least the hold music was marginally better. It sounded like an easy listening radio station—Christopher Cross or something. I clicked through some patient tasks on my laptop, though I was distracted by my own frustration.

It didn't help that I was dizzy that day. In addition to robbing me of creativity and motivation, dizziness sucked dry the tiny puddle of patience with which I had started the day. At last, I heard, "Thank you for your patience. You will now be connected with an agent. For quality assurance purposes, your call may be monitored."

To my great relief, a real, live person spoke. "Good day. Thank you for calling Phone Trees R Us Pharmacy. How may I help you?" I provided all my requisite numbers, told my tale of woe again ("and I arrived home expecting to see the box with my medicine on my front porch, but it wasn't there!"), and waited some more while the pharmacy tech researched my situation.

"It appears that your prescription was canceled," she finally said.

"What? Why would my prescription be canceled?"

"The old prescription expired, and your doctor has not sent in a new prescription," she explained. At least I think that's what she said. I struggled to understand her thick accent, imagining her far away— halfway around the world, quite possibly—trying to help me with my prescription refill. Maybe people who answer phones for these large companies are intentionally far away so that enraged patients don't try to track them down.

"Well, that's very interesting. Why didn't someone tell me that when we scheduled the shipment last week? Why didn't you all call me to tell me the prescription was canceled instead of just failing to deliver it?"

"We do apologize for the inconvenience, ma'am."

"Look, I know this isn't your fault, but can't you make an effort to contact me, to contact any of your customers who are expecting a delivery, when the prescription is expired?" I asked. "You all called me last week to arrange the shipment. Why did you call me if the prescription was invalid?" It felt a little weird to be doling out business advice, but this company needed it. "I mean, if I don't get my medicine, my health is at risk," I added for good measure. I wanted to go on to share that I was a parent of two little girls, that I needed to be able to take care of them, not to mention my patients, but I knew it was pointless.

"We apologize," the agent said again.

"So, what do I need to do now?" I asked. "Call my doctor?"

"Yes. Your doctor needs to send another prescription. Then we will contact you about the delivery of the medication."

I got the fax number that Dr. Reynard's staff would need to send in the refill, and I hung up.

"You've got one," Sara Maria said, referring to my first patient for the afternoon clinic.

"Do I have time for another short phone call?" I asked.

"I think so. It will take a few minutes for me to get her back to an exam room," Sara Maria said.

I found Dr. Reynard's office number in my phone and hit the call button. After multiple rings, a recorded message came on: "We are unavailable to answer your call at this time. Our office is closed for lunch. Please try your call again later." I couldn't even leave a message. I slammed down the receiver. And when I called a few hours later, after I had finished seeing patients, Dr. Reynard's office was closed.

CHAPTER 22

Up the Down Escalator

October 2010

A flicker of a memory. The mall? A subway station? My sister and I were playing on the escalator. We were what? Six and nine years old? We'd run up a few steps and pause as the escalator whisked us back down. We giggled, taking turns to see how far we could climb.

Since my diagnosis, my life felt like one endless escalator, carrying me down in the wrong direction. I was running up with fury, determination. I was lugging the kids, pulling patients with me, too. They were heavy. I was totally preoccupied with going up, and if I paused for a second, I lost ground.

At the clinic every day, I would sit in front of my laptop, clicking through tasks in the EMR at the end of each session of patient care—medication refills, lab results, notes from Kim about patients calling with questions. As I tried to address one issue, another task would appear. If I took ten minutes to call that patient with side effects from her antibiotics or to discuss her low potassium, two or three more assignments would pop up. And then I had e-mail, meetings, and stacks of home health orders and radiology results to review. In those rare moments of reflection, I worried about our productivity goals and tenuous grant funding. The escalator never stopped.

At home, my situation wasn't any better. Any patience I once had with the kids was gone. My family and friends helped as much as they could, but I still spent many long weekends alone with Ella and Clara. Often my dizziness seemed worse on our days alone together, and the kids could detect my scent of vulnerability. Sometimes they would take turns throwing a tantrum; other times, they would join forces in a scream-fest that caused exponential chaos.

One Saturday afternoon, after a relatively peaceful hour of play with large cardboard boxes, I sent the kids to their rooms for rest time. While Ella protested with a normal level of five-year-old rage, Clara reacted as if I'd suggested she jump into a cauldron of boiling garbage. But I wasn't deterred. I sent Clara to her room, holding the door closed for a few minutes while she endeavored to escape. Then I tiptoed back downstairs and pulled large brown cushions off the couch to use as props. I was going to do restorative yoga!

Clara, realizing that I was no longer holding her door closed, flew out into the hallway and down the stairs.

"Mommy, I have a really big spider in my room!" she shrieked.

"Oh no! Is it bigger than you?" I asked, placing a cushion on the floor near the built-in cabinet.

"No."

"Phew! I was getting worried," I said.

"But it's really big and scary."

I rolled out the yoga mat. "Okay, Clara. I'll come take a look, but then you need to stay in your room for rest time."

Clara agreed, and we climbed up the stairs together. She searched for the spider in the corner of her room, but all we could find were a few strands of an old web. I removed the web and agreed to leave her door open since she had calmed down.

I was calculating the hours until Don would come home and adjusting my iPod earbuds when Clara appeared in the living room again, this time requesting a box of toys at the top of her closet. Knowing that without my intervention she would stack stools, pillows, and chairs in a precarious tower to get down the box by herself, I again accompanied her upstairs.

"Okay, Clara, but I need to close your door this time. Remember, it's rest time. You don't have to sleep, but you do need to stay in your room," I said. "If you come out of your room again, I'm going to have to take away the box of toys."

Clara was furious when I closed her door, but she stayed in her room crying. To cover her angry sobs, I blasted cheesy eighties music on my iPod as I positioned myself on the mat with my feet on the cabinet for the restorative yoga pose, Legs Up the Wall. I smiled at the irony of the first song, "Heaven," by Bryan Adams.

Bang! Clara was throwing toys and books at her door.

I tried to ignore her as the piano music to a Phil Collins ballad began next on my iPod.

I heard further crashes as I tried to take deep, relaxing breaths and smiled at the sheer ridiculousness of the situation. "Against All Odds" seemed like the appropriate song to describe my thwarted attempts at self-care.

Bang, bang, bang. Clara was knocking rhythmically on the door.

I thought of Don's experience, years before, while working at the pediatric emergency room during residency. Don had examined a child with an unusual chief complaint (reason for visit): "possessed by the devil." After the familiar run of ear infections, broken arms, and skin lacerations, Don listened to the little girl's family explain that she made objects move without touching them and was cursed with other paranormal powers. ("Did you ask her to show you?" I'd asked. He had not). While Clara, so far, had not demonstrated supernatural tendencies, I, like the girl's family, wondered if an exorcist might help.

Five more breaths. I counted Clara's banging: six bangs for every one of my slow, steady breaths. I turned up the music, but I could still hear her pummeling her door with every hard object at hand. Her persistence was remarkable. I could only hope she would carry it with her into adulthood and apply it to more productive endeavors. At last, I got up, deciding not to risk further damage to the door.

"Rest time is over," I announced, opening Clara's door and assessing the floor of her room strewn with shoes, clothes, books, and every toy out of the box from the top of her closet. "Ella, you can come out, too."

Ella appeared in her doorway, glaring at me. I had thought she'd be happy to be done with rest time, but she sensed my irritation and was already reacting to it.

That evening, after fighting dizziness all day and struggling to restore Clara's room to a place where I could walk without risking a serious foot injury, I turned to my older child and said, "Ella, I'm not feeling very good, and I'm having a hard time. I need you to be extra helpful and cooperative. Can you do that?"

"No!" she said.

How have I failed to raise compassionate children? I read stories about kids giving their allowance to the Salvation Army, starting a lemonade stand to collect donations for the World Wildlife Fund, raking leaves for an elderly neighbor. Meanwhile, I couldn't get my daughters to put their plates in the dishwasher or carry in a bag of groceries from the car, even when I was struggling to put one foot in front of the other. I worried that they'd never learn to consider others' feelings and needs. I worried that, even worse, they would grow up with a sense of entitlement.

I'm not suited for motherhood, I thought. I have no illusions about my temperament. I'm not laid-back, patient, or flexible. I didn't expect to be the kind of mom who makes cookies—or nowadays, homemade hummus and fresh cucumber slices—for afterschool snacks. But I scolded myself when I tried to dodge a game of Go Fish. Moms were *supposed* to be engaged with their children, to spend hours each day playing with them, marveling in their development, cheerfully cleaning up messes, and shrugging off tantrums. *What is wrong with me?* I didn't like pretending to be a princess or a pirate. Broken dollhouse furniture and dirty socks on the kitchen table made me crazy. No wonder my children weren't helpful.

On the other hand, I knew I was internalizing an image of motherhood that was at once old-fashioned, unrealistic, and absurd. This vision was narrow and rigid. It would make anyone feel inadequate. I wanted to forgive myself, but during the children's meltdowns and moments of rebellion, I felt angry that I'd been so naïve—a victim of a societal conspiracy to convince happy-go-lucky couples to have kids.

I followed the racket to find Clara dumping out pieces of her train set and magnetic building tiles all over the living room floor. Again.

Deep breath. "Okay, little Destructor, it's time for your bath. Let's clean this up together, and then we need to go upstairs," I said, squatting down to sort out train tracks from the magnets.

"Don't listen to her!" Ella instructed her sister. I sent her to her room and carried Clara upstairs for her bath.

"If motherhood were a job, I'd resign now," I wrote in my journal that night. "Or I would have been fired." Of course, had I been their employer, I would have fired my kids. Persistent tardiness, failure to follow clearly articulated rules and policies, and insubordination were all grounds for termination.

I often told my patients who were stressed over a sick family member, "You can't take care of your mother/daughter/brother if you don't take care of yourself." It sounded like a cliché—you know, "Put your oxygen mask on yourself before helping others," as the flight attendants say. And it was sometimes impossible, maybe even leading to self-blame and a sense of failure.

But what I was really saying to patients who served as caregivers was "You matter. You deserve to be cared for, too." As I struggled with my children and my job, on top of my diagnosis, I had to remind myself to heed my own advice. Maybe I would have to live with dizziness, but I could take care of myself in other ways. I would have to try again to tackle my stress and get some distance from the kids.

An in-person restorative yoga class, rather than a self-directed session in my living room, was a treat and the exact opposite of the rest of my life: relaxing, slow, calm. Jess, who accompanied me one time, called it "a cross between a massage and a nap." Although I regretted my inability to properly relax (I planned my evening and crafted my mental grocery list during yoga), I always felt better afterward. My dizziness score for the day, which I tracked nightly in my journal, might improve, going from a five (indicating, per my own definition, that I was functioning at 50 percent of normal capacity) to seven (70 percent): an acceptable level, a passing grade. I could better tolerate the screams and barrage of five- and two-year-old demands that would engulf me as soon as I opened the door to my house.

Don was required to work a whole weekend in mid-October. I had learned my lesson and lined up our regular sitter to watch the kids on Sunday afternoon. I knew that by noon I'd be losing my patience. I wouldn't be able to play with Clara's "babies" any longer, and Ella's constant "What can I do?" line of questioning would grow so irritating that I would be tempted to flee. I would go to restorative yoga and emerge renewed and chill.

My usual teacher, Leslie, was out. The room was hot and stuffy as I lay my gray mat on the floor and gathered a huge stack of props—big purple bolsters, blankets, blocks, and my lavender eye pillow. Chrissy, the substitute teacher, was young and enthusiastic, almost bubbly. She had us take turns discussing our various issues—I said my big one was insomnia. Others complained of anxiety and back pain.

We didn't do the gentle warm-up I was used to but, instead, a breathing exercise in which we were instructed to move our hands from our legs to our hips to our shoulders to our back to our head and down again, taking deep breaths and hissing on the exhalation with each movement. "Head, Shoulders, Knees, and Toes." I thought of the song learned by every preschooler. Then we prepared for our first longer pose: a sideways twist that was fully supported by bolsters and blocks. Chrissy's detailed soliloquy describing the setup for the pose was accompanied by a chain saw as a tree trimmer went to work outside the window.

Once we were settled in our twist, Chrissy continued, "In restorative yoga, you are completely supported by the props. When your mind starts to wander, take your focus back to your breath." Her soothing voice reminded me of a massage therapist or preschool teacher, but it sounded contrived and was distracting.

Once we got into our second pose—Mountain Brook, which consists of lying flat with a blanket under your head and low back and a bolster supporting your legs and feet—I was ready for silence. Chrissy, however, was prepared with relaxation tips and a lecture about her twenty years of yoga and meditation practice. She must have started learning yoga at age six, I estimated.

"We tend to lose focus—our attention moves away from the breath to other things. That's what it's supposed to do. Just direct it back gently, with love, to the breath," she whispered. The chain saw shrieked, but she was unfazed. "You can ask for anything you want. Don't hesitate to tell me if the room is too hot or cold, or if you need a blanket."

I tried to shut her out. *Deep, slow breaths.*

"If you need to adjust any of your props, please do so. This is your time to be picky. Make sure you are completely comfortable. Adjusting a bolster or moving your arms a little can make a big difference sometimes."

The chain saw, which had stopped for a minute, roared again.

Chrissy turned on a white noise machine. It sounded like a staticky television with an occasional chirp from a bird.

Wow, this is almost as noisy as our house, I thought as Chrissy launched into a discussion of meditation and hand relaxation techniques: "Balance your hands, if they are outstretched, on your third and fourth knuckles. Not your second and third. The third and fourth are much better and provide more stability and relaxation."

By that time, I had succeeded in transferring any kid-related irritation I'd felt earlier that day to Chrissy. I was ready to stick my third finger right in her chatty face.

We moved into the next pose—*supta baddha konasana.*

"I'm going to go around the room now and ask each of you how you're doing. Please let me know what I can do to help you feel more relaxed."

"Are you okay? Can I get you anything?" Chrissy whispered to each person.

You can shut the fuck up, I wanted to say when she got to me. Instead, I said, "No, I'm fine." I even tried to change my mental tirade to something a little more polite, like "It's wonderful that you're enthusiastic about teaching, but could you please quiet down for just a bit?"

As we prepared for the last pose, I was overcome with rage. *She's ruined my only chance this whole week to relax! Should I leave? Would that be rude?* But I reeled myself back in. *This is a good challenge. Well maybe not a* good *challenge, but a chance to practice meditation in the face of distraction. Against all odds.*

Chrissy walked past me, putting away stray props. "Remember your breath," she was saying. "And let me know how to help you feel more relaxed. Remember, this is your time. You are taking care of yourself."

Okay, she is soliciting feedback. "Hey, thanks. Maybe . . . could we just have silence during this last pose?" It was the nicest I could muster.

"Uh, yeah, sure," she said. I detected a hint of annoyance in her voice.

"Thanks," I said, and awkwardly moved into the final position.

She kept her word. The harsh whine of the chain saw continued periodically, but the tree trimmers were winding down, too. *Okay, this is it: my final chance to settle down, to let go.* But I spent the next fifteen minutes regretting my request for silence almost as much as I regretted the absence of my usual calming, quiet teacher. I had upset Chrissy. I should have kept my mouth shut.

The chain saw and the class both stopped at 5:00 PM. I wasn't relaxed. I felt like I'd ordered cherry pie and been served turnip greens. Well, I had tried. The increasingly loud voice in my head, chanting, *You have to take care of yourself,* would have to be satisfied for now.

c⁓

A few nights later, I had my first MS dream: I was standing in the bathroom getting ready for work when I suddenly lost my vision. I staggered to the bed, but as I was about to call Don from the next room, I lost my voice. Curled up on my bed, unable to speak or see, I then realized I couldn't move.

Ella once told me that she thinks a nightmare is actually good because when you wake up, you feel happy that it's not real. I've often thought this was a wise observation for a child. But when I awoke from the MS nightmare, my relief was eclipsed by tremendous anxiety: I could go blind! I could wake up paralyzed!

When I went back for my next MRI, six months after my relapse, I was convinced that I would have multiple new white spots. *Surely the recent surge in dizziness was another flare. And the time during the summer when my legs felt weird and prickly for a few days? That had to be another exacerbation.* The image of that escalator came to mind again. Even though I was injecting my medicine as directed, running at the lake whenever I could, asking for and accepting help from friends, and going to restorative yoga, I knew MS—callous and cruel—might be there, ready to push me down the escalator at any moment.

Don had joined me this time, and we looked at the radiologist expectantly after the MRI, bracing ourselves for his verdict.

"Nothing new there or there," he said, scrolling through the films. "That lesion was there before—it's okay. And that one, too." He pointed to another white spot.

I waited, scrutinizing the black-and-white pictures of my brain, searching for white spots, or even worse, the dreaded, permanent black holes.

"What about that one?" I asked, pointing at a small white smudge.

"Nope, that was there before. We're only concerned about the new stuff," the radiologist answered.

He flipped through a few more pictures and stopped, turning back to face us. Don clutched my hand. "Good news," said the radiologist. "No changes. You're doing great."

I thought he must be wrong. "Really? But I've had symptoms. My dizziness is worse again. I had leg numbness a while back. And I can't sleep."

"Well, I can't help you with the sleep, and you've had the dizziness before. You may be stuck with that, but it's not because of MS progression. The MRI looks good today—and the MRI is a pretty good test," he reassured me.

I was so used to discouraging news that I hardly knew what to do with this information. I had, in some ways, been using MS as an excuse to lower my ambitions. I couldn't run a marathon—I had MS. I could never consider a different job—I'd lose my disability insurance. Adventurous travel would soon be off the table. I couldn't pursue more advanced training or a new career path. What would be the point?

Thinking about the future used to make me happy. I'd envision a family game of soccer in the front yard or biking together around the lake. Or I'd imagine exploring a far-off country with Don, ducking down side streets, daring him to try a spicy snack, getting lost on hikes and finding our way back to civilization. But with my diagnosis, I had started to let go of those dreams—and to plan for what I thought was the inevitable. I needed to save for an early retirement. I needed to pick up sedentary hobbies. When I couldn't climb stairs, I would move from my second-floor bedroom to our downstairs guestroom.

To others, I looked healthy. I didn't *look* like I had MS, whatever that meant. My mom had warned me early on that revealing my MS diagnosis would change the way others saw me. She was probably right, in some ways. But far more than that, MS had changed the way I saw myself. I was fragile. I was focusing on what I had lost, and even more, on what I thought I stood to lose.

But this? I didn't expect a stable MRI. It opened up new possibilities. I could plan summer hiking trips. I could go on longer runs—maybe even run a marathon. Okay, maybe a *half*-marathon. In a few years, when the kids were a little older, I might be able to take them on outings to the Barton Creek Greenbelt and play Marco Polo in the pool. I could think of ways to move beyond the clinic to a position where I could impact health care on a population level, allowing me to address some of the inequities that infuriated and frustrated me in my current role. Though I still needed to prioritize self-care and stress management, maybe I could imagine a cane-free future. Maybe I could revisit those goals I'd written off as impossible.

CHAPTER 23

From Clueless to Competent

January 2011

A driana came to the clinic for a well-woman exam, but I nixed plans for a routine physical when I saw her "positive review of systems." To nearly every intake question, Adriana—a new patient—had answered in the affirmative: "Yes, I have chest pain. Yes, I have headaches. Yes, I have back pain. Yes, I have abdominal pain." Especially in a young, otherwise healthy person, so many ailments noted on the review of systems often points to underlying depression, anxiety, or post-traumatic stress disorder. While I can't discount the reported concerns, identifying and addressing the core mental health issue is essential to resolving the other symptoms. As expected, she had also marked, "Yes, I have mood changes."

Adriana managed a small smile when I entered the room and introduced myself, but she oozed sadness. Her dark hair was tangled. Her eyes were red, and her cheeks were gaunt. I forgot my own troubles—finding someone to help with afterschool childcare, a tingling in two fingers that had just started—and I tried to unravel hers. Her mother had died ten months before—a devastating loss. Two weeks later, her boyfriend was stabbed as she, in her third trimester of pregnancy, stood nearby. He had lived, but the trauma had put her into labor. The baby was born via C-section—a healthy little boy. But she and her boyfriend weren't safe, and they decided to move to Texas from Mexico to be near her sister, who had accompanied her to the appointment.

Since her mother's death, Adriana had suffered panic attacks, anxiety, and total despair. She reported having hopelessness, poor sleep, crying spells, no appetite, no pleasure in activities, trouble concentrating, and no energy "nearly every day" on the Patient Health Questionnaire (PHQ-9), a common screening tool for depression. I tallied her answers: twenty-three out of a possible twenty-seven points. Severe depression. It may have been the highest score I'd ever seen. And she was already on high doses of Prozac, prescribed by a doctor she'd seen in South Texas.

The last question on the PHQ-9 concerned me the most. It asks how often, over the last two weeks, the patient has had "Thoughts that you would be better off dead or of hurting yourself in some way." Adriana answered, "More than half the days."

When a patient mentions suicidal thoughts, big red flags go up for me: This is an emergency. The stakes are high. I can't screw up. For a selfish instant, I feel some frustration as well, and regret that in prioritizing this patient, I'll be running late the rest of the session. But as

I sat with Adriana, I buried those concerns and my fears of making a mistake. I had an opportunity to help, a chance to make a difference. We needed a plan. I turned to her sister.

Her sister, who appeared organized and concerned, would be key to our safety contract, especially given her boyfriend's unpredictable work schedule. Adriana may not have a full support circle, and I hoped that with time she could build one. But she had one key person. That would have to be enough for now.

As I struggled to reduce my own anxiety about how to handle the situation, I moved toward Adriana and took her hand. "I am so sorry for what you've been through." I wished for the zillionth time that my Spanish was better. "You are going to feel better," I said. Then I repeated the words Don had said to revive me from despair after my spinal tap: "One of the worst things about feeling really bad is that you think you'll never feel better, but you will."

Although I didn't share my own story with patients who had depression, I could relate to their sadness, if not their situations. In college and again in medical school, I had struggled with a depression that had sapped my energy, appetite, and motivation. In fact, my neurologist, Dr. Reynard, had recently proposed antidepressants again for my continued irritability and insomnia, but I was resistant, wanting to avoid side effects and wary of adding more medicine to my daily routine. And next to someone like Adriana, I was as happy as an elf in Santa's workshop.

Adriana teared up again, and her sister handed her another tissue.

"Do you feel safe now, with your sister?" I asked.

"Yes."

"If you were going to kill yourself, do you know how you'd do it?"

"No," she said, shaking her head.

"You don't have a plan?"

"No."

Thank God. This will probably work. She didn't have a specific plan, and her sister could keep watch. It wasn't foolproof, but we didn't have a lot of other options.

"Good. Adriana, I am going to give you a prescription today, but I'm going to need to call a psychiatrist. Actually, I'm going to want you to see the psychiatrist." I couldn't say the word for psychiatrist in Spanish—*psiquiatra*. Adriana's sister corrected me about six times, and we all smiled a little. "Can you stay with your sister tonight and tomorrow? Then I'll try to get you an appointment with the counselor on Wednesday."

She nodded. I looked at her sister. "Can you stay with her and make sure she's okay?"

"*Claro.*" (Of course.)

Thank God for sisters. Mine would have done the same for me. I was certain.

My work was far from done, but I felt confident that I didn't need to send her to the psychiatric emergency room. I left to make the necessary calls. I was relieved to now have access to much-needed mental health services, thanks to our strengthened affiliation with the other local community clinics. I got some suggestions from the *psiquiatra* to adjust Adriana's medications, and she agreed to return later that week after I had her lab results and she had seen the counselor. I said, "*Adiós*" and gently closed the door. *She'll get better,* I thought. *We both will.*

⌒

Kim came to my office that afternoon looking distraught. Apparently, an angry patient was threatening legal action.

According to Kim, the patient had called to schedule her well-woman exam. But when our receptionist, Elizabeth, asked for a contact phone number—part of the standard procedure for scheduling appointments—the patient became irate.

"What the fuck? I'm not going to give you my number!" she'd screamed at Elizabeth. "Don't you know it's illegal to ask for an unlisted private number! Goddamn it! I'm going to sue your sorry ass!"

"I don't think she ever got her appointment scheduled, but I just wanted to let you know," Kim told me, after recounting the conversation.

"Wow, I'm sorry. That must have been horrible. But I've got to say, I don't think she has a very good legal case against us," I said.

"I mean, a *contact phone number?* If she got so worked up about that . . . Some of these people scare me," Kim said.

"Well, thankfully most of our patients aren't like that," I said, angry and irritated that Elizabeth, who was considerate and mild-mannered, had to endure such abuse.

Sara Maria interrupted us. "Mrs. Waller is here. She sure is a nice lady!"

Indeed. I smiled at Kim.

My next patient, Nancy Waller, was here for her second visit with me. Her case interested me more than most. For over two decades, she had lived with MS.

A friend had referred her to me from a social services nonprofit. "She has MS, and I know you know a lot about that," she'd said. "She has other health issues, too, but she lost her insurance about a year ago. She really needs a doctor."

Prior to my own diagnosis, I would have been overwhelmed to see a new patient with MS. It had been foreign and mysterious, with unfamiliar treatments, medicines with unpronounceable names, and the potential for catastrophic outcomes. But now I felt competent and curious. I knew the symptoms, the meds, the tests to order.

I assumed, when I first saw Mrs. Waller, that MS was the reason for her wheelchair. She was hunched over, her legs immobile and her left arm pulled up against her abdomen. But to my surprise, MS was the least of her worries and not the reason for her paralysis.

"I had a stroke," she said, her speech slurred, though I could still understand her. "I was active before that. I was hiking the Appalachian Trail, one section at a time."

Then one morning when she was home alone, she fell, presumably from the stroke.

"No one found me for a full day," she said. "I haven't been able to walk since."

"What about your MS?" I asked. "When were you diagnosed? What meds have you taken?"

"I've had MS for twenty years—maybe thirty," she said. "I've been on a lot of different medicines, but now I'm not on anything. The stroke is what really got me."

The reason for the stroke in this previously fit, fifty-five-year-old woman was unclear. She had seen a neurologist, and an array of tests looking for possible causes—a heart defect or arrhythmia, a blocked carotid artery—was normal.

During the two weeks between visits, I had done my homework. In reviewing Mrs. Waller's old records, I discovered that her MS had transformed from the relapsing, remitting form to secondary progressive MS, with worsening disability. Prior to 2017, when ocrelizumab became the first drug approved for progressive MS, no medicines were known to reduce MS-related disability in people like Mrs. Waller. (I even discussed her treatment options with Dr. Reynard.) Even now, treatments for both primary and secondary progressive MS are more limited than for the relapsing forms. But the bigger issue for Mrs. Waller was her stroke, which had left her severely disabled, though MS might have contributed to her limitations as well.

I also got back the results from Mrs. Waller's initial labs: no diabetes, no liver disease, no thyroid problems. But wait—her cholesterol numbers were among the highest I'd ever seen. A reason for her stroke? Perhaps.

Mrs. Waller greeted me like an old friend at our second visit. "Hello, Doctor! I'm glad to see you."

"I'm glad to see you, too. How's it going?" I asked.

"Pretty good. I've started taking aspirin, like you said."

"Great! That will help lower the risk of another stroke," I said. "And you know, your labs showed me that you need another medicine too to help prevent another stroke or a heart attack. Did you know your cholesterol is very high?"

"Really?" she asked. "I have a good diet. I don't eat sweets. I used to grow my own vegetables."

It sounded familiar. She took care of herself, exercised, lived a healthy, independent life. Yet she had been struck down, not only with MS, but with a stroke. You could do everything in your power. Eat your vegetables. Exercise. Get eight hours of sleep and find a four-leaf clover for good measure. So much for power.

"That's good to hear, and it's very important," I said, "but your cholesterol is definitely too high to control just with diet. We need to start a new medicine."

At least I had some explanation for what had happened, though I regretted finding it far too late. Her story reminded me that people with MS can, of course, get sick with other chronic conditions. Heart disease, certain autoimmune diseases, depression, anxiety, and yes, stroke all appear to be more prevalent in people with MS than the general population.[1] It's easy to lose sight of everything else—cancer screening, immunizations, cholesterol and diabetes testing—when something like MS is so dominant. For Mrs. Waller, I prescribed cholesterol medicine with the hope of avoiding further damage but knowing it would do nothing to restore what had been lost.

"Okay. I'll do what you say. Anything else?" she asked.

I reached out and squeezed her stiff hand. I didn't tell her about my own diagnosis because I wanted to keep the focus on her and would have been uncomfortable sharing too much personal information. But I felt a kinship with her and a regret that I hadn't seen her sooner, that no one had been able to stop her stroke.

"Well, there's not much we can do for your MS at this stage other than try to address your symptoms, but we'll do everything else we can to keep you healthy," I said. "We need to keep an eye on your blood pressure. It looks good today, but it was borderline last time."

I gave her a log to record her blood pressure readings and reviewed the potential side effects from the new cholesterol medicine. We briefly discussed her back pain, and then I bid her goodbye. She was complicated and would be a challenge to manage. I would have to make sure that MS and her stroke didn't eclipse other symptoms and problems that might arise, like high blood pressure. But, for a change, with this patient at least, having MS made me feel more confident, more prepared to take care of her.

CHAPTER 24:

Will You Hold My Hands When I Die?

January 2011

Ella's entry into kindergarten some months before had been marred by her excessive shyness and a tantrum that could only be stopped by the assistant principal's well-timed compliments of my daughter's sparkly new shoes. But at the midyear parent/teacher conference, I learned that my kindergartner who had melted down like the Wicked Witch of the West on the first day of school was "doing awesome."

"She is one of the best-behaved kids in class," her teacher continued.

Oh, thank God.

"She's even nurturing at times," her teacher added, smiling. "She'll encourage other kids by saying, 'Good job! You did great!'"

I smiled, too: progress. I remembered the Stages of Change model popular among therapists and health educators: after a period of Precontemplation, a person may start to think of quitting smoking, for example (Contemplation). Next, they may enter the stage of Preparation (throwing out ashtrays), followed by Action (quitting), and then Maintenance (staying quit).

For Ella, our Stages of Change model was more complicated: Parent Proposes Change (new camp, new school) led to Child Resists Frantically, followed by Parent Insists on Change (if not demoralized to the point of capitulation). The next stage, Child Again Resists Frantically, was followed by Parent Insists Frantically and then, astonishingly, Child Accepts Change and Seems Perfectly Fine. After the next stage, Parent Throws Away Applications for Kindergarten Boarding School, we would land in Maintenance until Relapse occurred.

I wished we didn't have to undergo the grueling Frantic Resistance phases with every new activity or schedule change, but I was elated that we were now in Maintenance with kindergarten. I could move on to the next item on my To Worry About List.

As for me, I was considering my own Stages of Change. For months I had been reimagining my future, contemplating the adjustments I needed to make to live with MS. Little by little, I had prepared and then taken action to quell my symptoms and reduce my stress. I weaned myself off sleeping pills that seemed to worsen my dizziness. A new laptop at work that I carried with me into patient rooms improved my workflow and efficiency.

The stable MRI had given me hope. I no longer felt like I needed to turn down opportunities to grow professionally and personally. I took on more responsibility at work, serving as interim director for another clinic, in addition to my own. We found a new dog and adopted her from the Austin Humane Society. The kids named her Clover. I let myself think about traveling, about running more—maybe a lot more.

e⁓

"Do dinosaurs like glue?" Clara asked from the back seat, interrupting my thoughts as I drove her to school one morning in mid-January.

"What?" I asked, turning down the radio to make sure I could hear her.

"Dinosaurs like glue?" she repeated, pulling on the broken shade I'd stuck on her car window to block out the direct sunlight. The shade had lasted less than three days with Clara before falling apart and becoming a mildly interesting toy for her.

"Well, they didn't really coexist, but I guess the dinosaurs would not have liked glue." I smiled. *Where did she come up with these questions?*

"Glue doesn't taste good," Clara said.

"No, it doesn't. Glue isn't for eating." *When had Clara been tasting glue?*

As Clara and I walked into her preschool, I smiled down at my tennis shoes. Until recently I had been one of the only mothers at drop-off who dressed up for work every day. Now I had ditched my black boots and flats. I had joined the other moms in tennis shoes and sweatpants at drop-off.

At least on Wednesdays, I had adjusted my schedule to stay home from work. It was a dramatic act—and uncharacteristic of my drill-sergeant mentality. The staff now functioned well without me, and my employers agreed that I could work slightly less than full time. It was a nod to self-care, an acknowledgment that a better work-life balance wouldn't magically happen. Although my other workdays became a little longer as a result, on Wednesdays, after taking Clara to school, I would go home.

I didn't relax on those days off. Turning into my driveway, I could feel heart palpitations. Desperate to pack in as much as possible, to feel a sense of accomplishment, I would attack my to-do list: e-mail, errands, emptying the dishwasher, phone calls, more e-mail. I would set the kitchen timer and clean up like I was competing in a track-and-field event. Or I might head straight to the computer to review patient-related tasks and prescription refills from home.

In medical residency—our intensive training program after medical school when we routinely worked eighty to one hundred hours a week—I remember one of our attending physicians telling us that we would never again have as much time as we did then. *Are you crazy?* I had thought. *I am not going to work these kinds of hours when I'm done with residency. No way.* But now, when I added childcare time together with work time, I was easily pushing one hundred hours a week.

Of course, taking the kids to the Austin Children's Museum and making cookies together could be more fun than assessing asthma severity or adjusting insulin. But playing Candyland and cleaning up dried paint and glitter after an arts and crafts extravaganza were not. And all these activities were overshadowed by thoughts of the patient lab results I needed to address, the endless piles of laundry, and the overflowing closets and drawers in our house begging to be organized. I knew that no matter what I did during my day off, I would feel rushed and frustrated that I couldn't fit in a week's worth of tasks into eight hours of free time (which is not the right term at all). I'm just programmed to fill every second with too much.

But I felt a little bit proud that I had worked more kid-free hours into my schedule. Jess had recently told me with a mixture of regret and amusement that her three-year-old had drawn a picture on their driveway with chalk of her too-busy dad. An impressive picture, the drawing had a head, eyes, ears, nose, mouth, and four extremities. But what caught Jess's attention was the unusually large ear on one side.

"Why is that ear so much bigger than the other one?" she had asked.

"That's not his ear," said her daughter, giggling. "That's Daddy's phone!"

I could imagine my kids would have drawn me physically attached to my computer. And that needed to change. Plus, I loved putting on sweats and wearing slippers on Wednesdays.

My need for that extra kid-free time at home was driven, in part, by Don's hospital schedule, which continued to include evening and weekend shifts. I liked to think that my Wednesday organization sessions meant that I was more present and available for the kids, especially when I had them to myself.

One evening, when Don was working at the hospital, I read two bedtime books to the kids. Then I flicked off the light and started to tell them the story of my first date with their father, nineteen years ago that very night.

"So, you know your dad and I met in Boston, but a couple months later, he came to visit me for the first time," I said. "He came on a bus to my college—Amherst. When he got off the bus, I thought, 'He's really tall, and he's cute.' I gave him a hug. Then we went out to dinner at the Lord Jeff Inn—"

Clara interjected, "Mimi dived?"

Huh? Where did that come from?

"Yes, Honey, Mimi died," I answered. Clara was the queen of non sequiturs, but this reference to my grandmother Mimi's death, just a few months before Clara was born, was particularly unexpected.

"Mocha dived?" she continued. Her persistence in using the word "dived" instead of "died" was endearing.

I pulled up the sheets around us and snuggled closer to her.

"Yes, Mocha died," I said. Clara hadn't known my grandmother, but the loss of our dog, Mocha, had been more real to her. "Don't you want to hear about my first date with your dad?" I was eager to change the subject.

But Clara persisted. "Why did Mimi dive?"

"Well, sweetie, she got old, and her body was worn-out," I said, kissing her head. Even with the light from the hallway, her face was in shadow. I couldn't see her expression.

"Everybody gonna dive?" she asked.

How could I answer this question for a three-year-old? It's so much worse than, well, anything. I told the truth, "Yes, everyone eventually dies."

She burst into tears. "NO!!!" she shouted.

Her reaction was absolutely appropriate. I was struck by the enormity of her realization. I was watching this tiny child learn the worst of life's secrets.

I tried to comfort her, but I was at a loss. *How do you put a positive spin on death?*

"Oh, sweet Clara, this is why we have to enjoy every day. Life is an incredible gift," I said, squeezing her with one arm and stroking her hair with my other hand.

"I gonna dive?" she asked.

"Not for a long, long time. You're going to live a long, happy life."

"No! I not gonna dive!" she screamed, terrified.

I tried to reassure her that she would not die until she was very, very old, but that only added to her panic.

"I don't want to get old!" she wailed.

Meanwhile, Ella was sitting next to us, calm and quiet. We had talked about the birds and the bees and the cycle of life. We had referenced death in conversation but had never discussed it so directly. I turned to her and reached out to rub her arm. "Ella, what do you think about all this?"

"I don't really think about it a lot," she said.

I patted her shoulder, worrying that she might be upset, too, but she seemed okay.

"The lion gonna dive?" Clara started again, fighting back more tears.

"I don't see any lions around here, but the lions will die, too," I said. Thinking that I could reassure her a bit, I added, "People and animals die so new babies can be born."

That didn't seem to placate her. She went on with her questions, asking if Ella would die, if Daddy would die. I tried to dodge a few questions, but mostly I went on answering, so awed by the whole experience of this massive, awful realization for her. I couldn't come up with a worthy distraction. Plus, I was torn between getting it all out there versus pushing it aside, knowing that she might be wondering and worrying alone.

She seemed to feel a bit better when she asked if our house would die, and I told her it would not. Unfortunately, Ella disagreed, interjecting that even the house would someday turn into dust.

"Our house is strong and sturdy," I said, without exactly conceding to Ella. "Our house will be here for a long, long time."

Clara then asked if she would keep her hands when she died.

"Yes, you can keep your hands."

"Will you hold my hands when I dive?" she asked.

I brushed back my own tears at that little wish, and I squeezed her small hands.

Surprisingly, she went to bed easily after that, saying she wanted to stay in our house, and was relieved to hear that her room wouldn't die.

I just wanted to keep holding her, but I knew she needed to sleep. I went downstairs and called Don.

"Poor little girl!" he said, after I recounted our conversation. "I wish I could have been there."

"Me too. I don't even know why she's talking about this. I mean, Mocha died months ago, and Clara fortunately hasn't experienced any other losses," I said.

Maybe it was the damn movies! As Don and I became familiar with the plots and characters of popular children's movies, we were startled and amused to see that nearly all of them either start with the premise that one or both parents have died or that a parent is ill or absent. Four-letter words will prompt at least a PG rating, but parental death is apparently an acceptable topic for even the youngest kids. Think of every Disney movie you've ever seen: *Cinderella, Bambi, Finding Nemo, Aladdin, The Little Mermaid.* All heroes and heroines are orphans or, at best, raised by single parents after the death of the other parent. I had been irritated when I had watched *The Lion King* a couple of months before my conversation with Clara about death. Not only did the animals call one another "stupid," but Simba, the hero, watched his father die and was implicated in the death. I talked to the kids about this common theme in children's movies; we even joked about it. When *Frozen* came out a couple years later, Ella and Clara already expected the parents to die.

"Yeah, the parents were in a shipwreck and never heard from again," Ella explained to me after returning from the theater with her dad. "Of course they died. It's a kids' movie!"

c⁓

Clara's discovery, the stark reality of death—combined with the uncertainty of my own future—reinforced my change in attitude. While I had reminders of life's brevity on a regular basis at work, I had learned to compartmentalize and shove it aside. We live and die. So it goes. Too bad. But could I really be that blasé?

I had always lived with uncertainty. We all do—and with an awareness of our mortality. We try to push it out of our minds. We don't like to admit how powerless we are to predict and control our destiny. Clara provided a reality check. She responded to the notion of death with the horror it deserved. And MS, though it was unlikely to shorten my life substantially, added an extra dose of uncertainty about the kind of life I would lead and the limitations I would face. Unwelcome as it was, my illness was a wake-up call for me to figure out what was important, stop waiting for the right moment to do more, and do it now.

CHAPTER 25

The Renovation

May 2011

My clinic was undergoing a renovation. A local foundation had accepted our grant request to remodel, allowing us to create two more exam rooms, a reconfigured front-desk space and waiting room, and a much-needed closet. Large blue plastic sheets and makeshift walls shielded our view, but the banging of hammers and screech of saws permeated the clinic. Reduced to only two functioning exam rooms, we had cut back our schedules. And when someone ran late, the resulting domino effect impacted everyone. Patients sat next to boxes in the temporary waiting room and listened to drills while waiting for their appointments.

Despite the inconvenience, I was excited about the remodel, especially the two new exam rooms. Terri and another nurse practitioner, Joy, would increase their hours from part-time to full-time. We could improve our workflow and see more patients. It was a little metaphorical for me, too: like my shifting perspective and changing priorities, the clinic was evolving.

I was embarrassed about the state of the clinic–construction zone when I saw my new patient, Adam. But he was too miserable to care about stacks of boxes in the corner of the exam room and the occasional shriek from the power tools.

"The pain started, like, about two weeks ago," he said. "Well, I'd been having pain before that, but about two weeks ago it seems like it kind of flared up, and it just keeps getting worse."

Adam was in his mid-twenties. He was new to the clinic, heavy set with premature hair thinning, wearing an old flannel shirt. I could tell he was having serious abdominal pain as he grimaced and shifted his position on the blue plastic and metal chair in the corner of the exam room. He clutched the right side of his abdomen as he talked, breathing rapidly.

"I've also been throwing up. It's usually just in the morning, but yesterday it happened a couple times during the day. There was some blood, too." He paused again, moving forward in his seat a little. I noticed a hole in the toe of his tennis shoe. "My girlfriend is pregnant, and I haven't been able to work for the last two weeks. I'm pretty sure I'm gonna get laid off," he said.

I questioned him further about the vomiting and asked all the requisite questions: Can you describe the pain? Is there anything that makes it better or worse? Is it constant, or does it come and go? Do you have any other symptoms, like fever, diarrhea, constipation, burning with urination?

As I listened to his heart and lungs, I was thinking of my differential diagnosis. *An infection? An ulcer? Pancreatitis? An obstruction?* Cancer was unlikely at his age, and appendicitis would have declared itself by now. Though he had moved slowly getting onto the exam table, he nearly bolted off when I touched his abdomen.

"Oh God! Stop!" He jerked to the side as I gently probed the right upper quadrant of his belly, trying to assess the size of his liver.

"I'm sorry. I'll stop," I said, moving back from the table and dropping my hands to my sides. "I'm sorry to hurt you. I can tell you're having really terrible pain." I sat back down on my stool, rubbing my hands again with more white foam sanitizer.

"Oh, I can't take this!" he moaned, rolling from side to side on the exam table, slowly sitting up again, and looking more distressed than ever.

"Adam," I said. "I don't know exactly what's going on with you, but I think this pain is bad enough that you need to go to the ER."

"Oh God, I was afraid you'd say that," he said, putting his hand to his forehead. "My girlfriend has been telling me to go for days. I did go one time, but I waited for three hours and never got back to see anyone, so I left."

"Is this the worst pain you've ever had?" I asked. This was a red-flag question. A "yes" got my attention, indicating a possible emergency and need for surgery. The associated vomiting, especially with blood, was another big concern.

"Oh, for sure," he said, tears coming to his eyes. "I can't go though—to the ER, I mean. I'm already behind on rent. I can't do it."

I hated these conversations. They indicated a failure: my failure to diagnose and help him and the system's failure to provide an affordable way for him to get the care he needed. Moral distress at its finest. In other parts of the world, an ER visit would have been inexpensive or even free. If I needed to go to the ER—if my MS left me suddenly paralyzed or if I had a bad fall on the running trail—I would only have to pay a hundred-dollar co-pay. My insurance company would pay the rest. But because Adam was uninsured and made just a little too much money to qualify for the Medical Access Program, he could be stuck with a bill that might exceed the yearly rent on his apartment. This scenario was all too familiar. The injustice was infuriating.

"It's an unfair system," I said.

"Yeah, I've really been trying. I mean, I want to take care of my girlfriend. I want to be a good father, you know, once the baby is born. Now I'm just, like, stuck," he said. "I was supposed to get insurance at work if I stayed long enough, but now I can't work."

Right. He was stuck. "Adam, I know it's expensive to go to the ER, but you don't have a choice. Look, I think you need a CT scan, and I can't get that done for you quickly. You may even need to have surgery."

"No!" he moaned. "You said you didn't know what it is, and now you think I need surgery?"

"I don't know. Your symptoms don't fit the pattern of appendicitis, but if it was something like that, you would need surgery. I'm sorry. I wish I could tell you. I just don't know," I said.

I wheeled my stool over to the box of tissues on top of my supply cabinet and handed him the whole box. Tears were flowing down his cheeks, and he was rocking slightly, still massaging his abdomen with one hand. I touched his other arm, just above the elbow. "Hey, I think you're going to be okay. You seem like you're otherwise pretty healthy, but you need to get this taken care of now. You've been having pain too long."

He nodded, wiping his eyes with a tissue.

"The ER has to see you, even if you can't pay. It's a law," I said.

"They can work out a payment plan with you, but that's not nearly as important as getting you better."

He nodded again, and I helped him off the exam table and back to the chair, where he picked up his scratched cell phone.

"I'll write a note for you to take to the ER. I'll also call the ER and let them know you're on your way. I'd like to see you back on Friday," I said, standing up to leave.

"Yeah, okay," he said.

I returned to my office, feeling empty, helpless. As a doctor for the uninsured, I was inclined to do everything I could to keep people out of the emergency room. I was always hearing news stories of ERs crowded with uninsured patients, coming in for nonemergencies because they had nowhere else to go for care, crowding out the people who really needed help. I remembered the story of a teenager who called EMS to go by ambulance to the ER for a refill of acne medicine. In residency, I worked in the ER. People came in demanding pain medicine. Some showed up with simple problems—a cold, an ear infection—that would be better handled in an outpatient clinic. Some came in just because they were lonely.

It was easy to blame those who misused the ER—easier to place blame than to own the problem, improve access, provide health care to everyone regardless of income. I didn't have all the answers, but in my experience, most people didn't go to the ER for fun. Thanks to a federal law, the Emergency Medical Treatment & Labor Act, passed in 1986, hospitals that accept Medicare (and most do) can't turn away anyone without assessing and stabilizing them. But emergency care is expensive, and uninsured patients often receive exorbitant bills. The ER was usually my last resort.

Every few weeks or months, I saw an uninsured patient with a true emergency who refused to go to the ER. Usually, the reason was financial. Sometimes, if my patients couldn't be convinced, and I was worried about a life-threatening condition, I would scribble a statement for them to sign, saying that they accepted the risk to their health for failing to follow medical advice. In those cases, I would still do my best to treat them, ordering the necessary labs and other tests, but I always worried about the delay. I could sometimes get STAT labs in a few hours, but getting an urgent radiology test—which had to be done at a different facility—was difficult, if not impossible.

Plus, our clinic wasn't equipped to support patients as they waited for test results. We couldn't start an IV, consult a surgeon, or perform an ultrasound. A patient had to be sent home. Then, if a test came back confirming a true emergency, Kim and I would be left trying to track down the patient to convince them that really, now, the ER was the only choice. I was relieved that Adam agreed to go without too much resistance. And I hoped the ER doctors would make a concerted effort to help him. Like the cheap, kid-friendly restaurants we frequented, the service in the ER could be a little spotty.

⌒

I knew immediately when they started gluing in the floor tiles one afternoon the following week. The smell was worse than my car on a hot day when I'd left my yogurt container from breakfast inside. We had planned for the work to start after we had finished with patients for the day, but I was running behind. One of my patients—Tiffany— had called in the middle of the afternoon reporting suicidal thoughts.

"Her boyfriend just got out of jail—the same guy who burned down her house," Kim had reported when I came out of an exam room. "She picked him up from jail—this was last week. That night he beat her up again. She says he dragged her by her hair, and she broke two ribs when he knocked her against a door."

Kim followed me to my office. I was between patient appointments, and I collapsed into my desk chair. Tiffany had worn us all out. Her story was tragic and heartbreaking—one of the worst I'd ever heard. Yet I was short on empathy. A few years younger than me, Tiffany seemed to resist all our efforts to help. She showed up for her appointments only half the time, yet she called Kim every other week with a similar story from her soap-opera life. She would disappear for months, and then resurface, sometimes walking in without an appointment, angry at everyone, demanding to be seen. But I reminded myself of her wretched abuse history and mental health problems. In her position, I would be angry, too. I took a deep breath and summoned patience to problem-solve with Kim.

"Is she still with this guy now?" I asked.

"No, he's back in jail," Kim explained. "But she was crying on the phone saying she wants to overdose on her psych meds."

"Is she still on the phone now?"

"Yes, she agreed to stay on hold," Kim said. "I told her not to hang up or I'd have to call the police."

"Well, let's see if we can avoid that. Let's call her case worker and see if they can send their mobile crisis unit over to assess her," I said.

While Kim kept her on the phone, I tracked down the case worker. At some point, Tiffany had qualified for disability benefits, due to serious mental health problems. I was thankful that she had Medicaid coverage as well as a case worker from the local mental health center. Multiple calls, phone trees, and accidental hang-ups put me thirty minutes behind schedule, but I finally reached the right person.

"I just talked to Tiffany this morning, and she seemed okay," she said.

"Well now she's threatening suicide with a specific plan to OD. My nurse has her on the phone in the other room. Can y'all get someone out to check on her?"

The case worker seemed as exasperated with the patient as I was, but she agreed to have the mobile van pay her a visit.

I walked back to Kim's office to give her a thumbs-up. "They are on their way."

Kim acknowledged me with a nod. "And when is the court date?" she asked Tiffany over the phone. A loud hammer was pounding nearby, and Kim had her finger in one ear so that she could hear Tiffany through the other. "Okay, well, you're safe now. . . . Bad timing . . . right."

Kim explained to Tiffany that the mobile van was on the way and hung up the phone. "I think I talked her off the ledge, but man, is she a mess!" she said. "You know her godfather—the one who abused her—is sick now, and she's been helping to take care of him."

I was exhausted and struggling to remain compassionate. We all were trying to help Tiffany. I later learned about Adverse Childhood Experiences (ACEs)—things like experiencing or witnessing violence, having a parent addicted to drugs, losing a family member to suicide—that have a negative, long-lasting impact on health and life opportunities. Tiffany would need all fingers on both hands to count her adverse experiences. Her wounds were deep, and we didn't have the means to fix her.

"I don't even know what to say at this point. . . . Did she ever go to Safe Place like we discussed last time?" I asked, referring to the local shelter for victims of domestic violence.

"She says she tried but didn't have money for gas or something," Kim said.

"Okay, well, thanks for all your help. I don't think she'll show up, but of course you can offer her an appointment," I said. Then I hurried back to my office and logged back into the EMR.

I raced to catch up and gave thanks to the God of Small Favors when my fifth patient was a no-show. When the glue fumes seeped under the exam room door, I was almost finished with my last appointment.

"Okay, Mr. Sanchez," I said in Spanish. "I've just sent your prescription refills to the pharmacy. Please remember to try to get back to walking every day. That, and your medicine, should help your blood pressure."

"Yes, I'll try," he said, standing up to leave.

"Sorry about all the noise today," I added.

"*No importa*" (It doesn't matter), he replied, reaching out to shake my hand, polite as always.

"Next time the clinic should look a lot better," I said, bidding him goodbye.

I had planned to stay for another hour or so to finish up my patient notes, but within just a few minutes the whole clinic had been infused with a poisonous odor. My dizziness, thankfully, was mild that day, but I knew it would get worse if I stayed. Even Terri, who practically lived at the clinic, was packing up to leave.

"Have a good weekend," I said to Terri. "Hopefully by Monday this place won't smell like a toxic waste dump."

The glue odor had faded by the following week when Kim and I met with the renovation project manager.

"We should be finished by the end of the month," he assured us. "We're on target with the floors. We have a little more painting to do, but the noisiest parts are all finished."

I was relieved that we would soon be able to return to our regular schedule. The productivity numbers were in for the last two months. We were behind, as usual.

At a recent meeting of physicians and administrators from multiple community clinics, an EMR consultant from the East Coast had come to talk to us about another much-anticipated EMR upgrade. "As a family physician, I generally see thirty-six patients a day, keep up with all my documentation, and finish at five o'clock," she told us.

I looked at the person next to me—a seasoned internist. "No way," I whispered. "Thirty-six patients?" I couldn't see half that number without rushing all day and staying late to finish my notes, well into the evening. With more support staff, a better EMR, and a well-resourced patient population I would have been faster. But thirty-six patients a day?

"And I guarantee I could get at least seventy percent of you up to that same level of efficiency and productivity," the consultant added.

I stared at her. I would feel proud indeed to see just twenty patients a day and finish my notes by 5:00 PM.

"It's just not possible!" I said to Terri later that day.

"Obviously, quality of care would suffer—a lot," she said. "But I couldn't even provide poor quality of care and see that many patients."

"I wish I could watch this doctor in action," I said. "It would be like going to the circus, like watching the superhuman feats of acrobats and lion tamers. Plate spinners! It's almost as incredible as someone managing a household with four or five kids!"

Doctors are often asked and expected to do the impossible: find explanations for symptoms that don't make sense or solutions to problems that stem from desperate living situations and personal crises far beyond our control. The productivity demands were also unreasonable, and they continue to be so. A simulation study published in 2022 estimated that a primary care provider, with an average-sized patient panel, would need to work almost twenty-seven hours a day to deliver all guideline-recommended preventive, chronic disease, and acute care. A well-functioning team working alongside that provider can cut the time substantially, to just over nine hours,[1] but many practices lack the skilled (and expensive) staff support—counselors, dietitians, nurses, physician assistants—needed to off-load from the doctor.

Although I volunteered to be trained by the consultant to be more efficient, the clinic administration was focused instead on the EMR upgrade, and other efficiency training never occurred. I was doubtful that the EMR upgrade would improve our productivity, but with the completion of the remodel and the arrival of a new part-time doctor, I knew we would be able to see more patients.

One afternoon, the construction workers tore down the temporary walls to reveal, like magic, a new clinic. I walked out of the conference room, and I wanted to start clapping. The hall, which had been blocked off for two months, was suddenly twice as long. The ledge for the new checkout window at the new front office was visible from the door of my office. We had gone from five to seven exam rooms, and at last we had a closet! Sara Maria, Elizabeth, Terri, and the other staff joined Kim and me for the tour. We couldn't pop open champagne bottles, but we cheered and laughed in celebration. It was clean and fresh with white paint and no clutter (yet). We opened to patients the next day.

CHAPTER 26:

Happy to Be Wrong

September 2011

ennifer, a new patient, came to see me at the clinic in late September. She was accompanied by her partner, an athletic woman who had once seen me for a minor knee issue and who I'd since spotted running at the lake. They were both in their thirties and had moved to Austin a year earlier. I greeted them, and we sat together in one of the new exam rooms so Jennifer could tell me about her migraines.

"My headaches have been a little worse over the past few months," she said. "I used to get them just every once in a while, usually when I didn't get enough sleep. Now I get them at least every week or so." She tucked a lock of mid-length brown hair behind an ear and then dropped her hands into her lap. As she spoke, I typed along in the EMR. (I still hated the EMR, despite the upgrade, but I was now well acquainted with its eccentricities and able to keep up.)

"Besides being more frequent, have the headaches changed at all?" I asked, intentionally looking up from my laptop to make eye contact.

"Not really," she said.

"Have you had any other new symptoms? Any visual changes, numbness, or weakness?"

She shook her head, but her partner jumped in. "You've talked about weakness a couple times, remember?" she said to Jennifer.

"You know, that's right. It's not all the time, but sometimes I do feel like my legs are a little weak." We both looked down at her feet, her beige flats and my black ones. "I've had some back pain, too, every once in a while," she added.

"Did you ever injure your back?" I asked.

"I was in a car accident a couple years ago. I've had pain off and on since then," she said.

"Have you ever had an MRI? I'm not sure you need one, but . . ."

She nodded. "Yes. I had a brain MRI back when we were in Alabama. I never got the results. I think they just did x-rays on my back when I had the accident, and it was okay."

I examined Jennifer, including strength testing of her legs—all normal. It was reassuring, though I recalled my own normal exam when my first MS symptoms appeared. We talked about starting a medication to prevent migraines, and she signed a release to get her old records sent to us. I also gave her a handout with some stretches for her back and referred her to physical therapy.

I didn't think much about her until a couple weeks later when Kim brought me the MRI report. With the skills and persistence of an investigative reporter or FBI agent, Kim had traced the MRI to an obscure radiology office in Alabama. I scanned the two-year-old report:

"white matter changes." A few years before, I would have had no idea what those changes could mean. Now I felt an anxious chill.

"Hmm. Was anything else done to work her up for MS?" the neuroradiologist asked, when I called to discuss the case over the phone.

"It doesn't sound like it," I said. "She says no one ever gave her the MRI results, and then she lost her insurance and never followed up."

"Well, it's not clear-cut," he said. "But it is suspicious for MS. What are her symptoms now?"

"Back pain, which she and I both thought was related to the car accident, and leg weakness, which would, of course, be more typical of MS. Her exam is normal. I was going to repeat the brain MRI and also get a spinal MRI."

"Yes, that's what I'd recommend," he said.

I called Jennifer myself to tell her the plan. Usually I would have had Kim call, but I felt a connection with this patient, like I'd just discovered we might be related.

I told Jennifer that the old MRI showed some changes that could be from her migraines. Her back pain could be related to the accident. But I also told her we couldn't rule out MS. I hated to burden her with an uncertain diagnosis, remembering the many times I'd faced similar situations: "I don't know what is causing your double vision and dizziness," or "We don't know if and when you'll relapse." I emphasized that we can't fully explain many things in medicine, and I knew better by that point not to make predictions.

"I'm glad you've got coverage with the Medical Access Program because it should cover most of the cost of the MRIs," I explained, after reviewing the old report with her. "The new MRIs will help a lot for us to understand what's going on."

"Okay, Dr. Doggett. What should I do until then?" she asked. Her voice was steady and calm. Fake calm, maybe? Hopefully, I could provide some reassurance.

"I'm glad you're asking. It's hard to have to wait for an answer to explain what's going on," I said. "For now, go ahead and make the appointment with the physical therapist for your back and start doing the exercises on the handout I gave you."

"Okay, I will."

"Let me know if any new symptoms develop, and I'll see you back after the MRI," I said. "I know it's a lot to take in, but we'll take this one step at a time and try to get some answers for you."

As I hung up, I wondered if I was being too paranoid. MS was on my radar all the time. I now knew it could present in so many ways, and I didn't want to miss it. But I knew I was biased, which I guess was inevitable. And I wondered, *Am I reading too much into this old MRI report? Am I getting worked up over nothing, creating anxiety, wasting everyone's time? Or maybe I'm about to make an important diagnosis that has been overlooked for years.* I hoped, for the patient's sake, that my hunch was wrong.

⌒

At a baby shower that weekend, a friend introduced me to another guest whose sister had MS. It was . . . awkward: "Oh, hi there, Miranda. This is my friend Lisa. I don't think she'll mind my sharing that she has MS, like your sister," my friend said as if she were pointing out that we'd both gone to the same college or enjoyed gardening. She had the best of intentions, and I loved her for that, but amid the talk of babies, onesies, diaper genies, and childcare options, it felt uncomfortable. Out of place. An unexpected sting.

Then my friend left me with this stranger, and we started to apologize to each other. "I'm sorry to hear that," we said almost in unison. Surrounded by happy friends exchanging baby advice, I assumed, at least, that she would share a hopeful story.

I asked, "So, how's your sister doing?"

"Pretty terrible, actually," the woman told me. "She's having a lot of symptoms—balance problems, word-finding difficulties."

I stopped smiling. "That's awful."

"Yeah, it's really unfortunate. She's kind of dropped out of life."

She seemed concerned, not overly so. But *I* was concerned. This was just one person we were talking about—I knew that. But she had the same disease and maybe she was just a little further on the path. Most of the people I'd met with MS since my diagnosis were doing well, but then again, I wouldn't encounter the ones who had "dropped out of life." I didn't want to be one of those people. I had to ask more questions. I needed to make sure that this sister we were discussing was nothing like me. I felt a little guilty probing, trying to satisfy my own agenda and curiosity. But I was acting out of fear, trying to gather what I needed to protect myself—a human reaction.

"How long has she had MS?" I asked.

"Nine years, I think. She's thirty-eight now."

My age, basically.

"The incontinence is really upsetting her. She has to wear adult diapers now. She doesn't want to go out anywhere," she continued.

Could I be looking at a homebound existence in a few years? I was sick thinking about it. "I'm so sorry," I said. And I was. But that didn't stop me from prying a little further. "What medicine is she taking?" I asked.

I wanted her to say that her sister didn't take medicine, that she believed in homeopathy or saw a shaman for treatment. That she insisted on only wearing green or eating foods that began with the letter R. Instead I learned that she took the same medicine I hoped would save me from disability and despair.

"I guess it's just really variable. MS, I mean. . . . You know, how MS . . . how it affects different people," I stuttered.

"Yeah, well, it's good you're doing well," she said.

I made an excuse to get a snack. I had heard enough.

Kim brought me Jennifer's new MRI report as soon as it arrived on the fax machine, a couple weeks after our phone call. "It looks okay," she said. "See what you think."

Turning my chair to face her, I took the paper from Kim and scanned the report: "Impression: Stable white matter changes, consistent with chronic migraines."

"Oh, thank God. It's not MS," I said, relieved that this pleasant young woman, who lacked financial resources, was spared. I had never been so happy to be wrong. We already knew Jennifer had migraines, and we could deal with that. An MS diagnosis in an uninsured patient, even one enrolled in the Medical Access Program, would have created significant challenges. Obtaining the expensive specialty medications and finding a qualified neurologist would have been no small matter, and of course the emotional toll of the diagnosis was all too familiar to me.

I rejoiced for Jennifer. She was going to be okay. But I still felt shaken by the story of my new acquaintance's sister. After a few months of modest improvement, my dizziness seemed worse again, and I felt vague leg numbness and tongue tingling. *Am I going to end up like the hermit sister, isolated, hopeless, afraid to leave the house?* MS was so random. *Life* was so random.

"I'm thinking about her again," I admitted to Don that night as we were getting ready for bed.

"Who?"

"That woman from the baby shower," I said, washing off my toothbrush. "I told you. . . . She has that sister with MS. You know, the one who 'dropped out of life'?"

"Oh yeah," he said. "Are you worried because you think that's going to happen to you?"

"Well, kind of. I mean, she's on the same treatment. . . ."

Don interjected, "That's *not* going to be you. There are some people like that, but there are a lot of people who aren't."

"I know, but, like in eight or nine years—"

"That's not going to be you," Don said again. "I know it won't be. You're doing everything you can to stay healthy, and even if you can't do everything you used to, I know you. You'll find a way to get around it."

Maybe he was right. Perhaps, even if I faced similar limitations, I could choose a different response. Mobility issues, incontinence, pain, visual loss, other new MS symptoms—they sounded awful, and yet . . . I could tackle those challenges. Never, ever would I drop out of life.

"And remember," he said. "Dr. Reynard said new medicines are being developed right now. Didn't he say the meds would get better before you get worse? If you relapse again, there will be something else."

Hope. We had that, too.

I decided to try yet another approach to address my dizziness: visual therapy. The physical therapist I had seen the previous year recommended this alternative when the vestibulo-ocular reflex exercises failed to help. I had put it off, but I finally decided I was ready to try something else. While I didn't want to perseverate on my symptoms, I also needed to know that I wasn't giving up. Even as a child I was told by various eye doctors that my eyes weren't "well coordinated." With a bit of effort or sometimes when I was tired, my eyes would move in different directions. Maybe visual therapy made sense.

Don came with me to the first appointment. It started out normal enough, with a comprehensive eye exam and testing with various lenses and eye patches. But the optometrist's conclusions were weird.

"You've got a leftward head tilt and difficulties with certain eye muscles," she said. "But it's complex and doesn't really fit into a neat package. I do think that our eye training program might help, though."

It was expensive, unconventional, and not covered by insurance, but I began weekly in-office eye-training sessions and daily exercises at home that were even more peculiar.

I started out learning to better coordinate and control my eye movements, practicing by slowly tracing the outline of objects—a chair, a window frame, someone's profile—with my eyes. I then learned to use props, like a three-dimensional vectogram that, in my case, consisted of two almost identical transparent cards that slid on top of each other, with letters in boxes connected by lines. I wore 3D glasses as I stared at the vectogram, training my eyes to line up the letters, even though they were separated on the cards. Another exercise required a ball that dangled from a string. I had to follow it with my eyes as it swung like a pendulum or moved in a circle around my head.

For one of the main exercises, I wore big, black-rimmed glasses and stared at a card with two columns, one with green circles and the other with red circles that looked like Life Savers. My job was to try to make the two circles converge in the middle. I had to concentrate, and my eyes would almost cross, or sometimes I'd see double. The circles would move back and forth, refusing to come together. But then, if I stayed calm and patient, I would succeed in bringing them to meet in the middle, forming a new gray circle.

"Do you think it's helping?" Don asked a couple months after I started the program. He was watching me as I sat in bed with the black glasses on, squinting at the card with the Life Savers.

"I don't know, but at least I'm trying something," I said. "And actually it does seem like I'm not having as many dizzy days now."

"That's good," he said. "If nothing else, you do look pretty cool with those glasses."

I knew the whole thing might be a huge waste of time and money. My insurance company, of course, would refuse to cover it, despite my pleas and appeals. But I wanted to overcome my dizziness, and I was out of options when it came to traditional treatments.

After several months, it was either helping or I had succumbed to the placebo effect and thought it was. Perhaps it didn't matter.

Driving to work one morning after a visual therapy appointment, I saw a homeless man as I was turning from 15th Street onto the IH35 access road. I often took that route to work, and I recognized some of the people from time to time who staked out a spot on that corner. I didn't think I'd ever seen this guy before, though. He was short and unshaven, wearing a dirty white shirt, baggy jeans, maybe fifty years old.

CHAPTER 27

You Win Some, You Lose Some

January 2012

Andy was back. And he was drinking.

"What happened?" I asked.

"I don't know exactly," he said. "One minute I was fine, and the next I was back at it." He was disheveled. His speech was slurred. My heart was breaking.

"Did something happen to set you off?" I asked.

"I don't even remember," he said. "I talked to my brother. That's never a good thing, but I don't know what did it."

I knew this could happen. I'd always known it. I'd almost expected it, especially when he missed a visit with me months earlier and didn't return our calls. Yet I had hoped so much for him to make it, to stay sober, to have a life again. I'd wanted him to fulfill his dream of becoming a counselor to help other people overcome substance abuse. He had been so close.

Andy wanted to be detoxed again. "I'm committed. I know there's a risk, but I just have to," he said.

"What's going to be different this time?" I asked.

"I don't know. I just—I have to try again."

So, try again we would. We were still stuck with no other options. No safer inpatient detox, no rehab center, no addiction medicine physician. Our clinic had a part-time counselor I could refer to now, but she wouldn't detox him, and she only came one day a week. We had to get him sober first. And I still wanted him to go to AA.

"I've been a couple times," he said. "It's just not for me."

"But each group is different. It's free, and there are meetings all over the city," I protested.

"Yeah, I'll think about it."

As with many of my patients, as with my own MS, I would try to balance hope with a need to protect myself from disappointment. Again, I feared for his safety. But we had succeeded before, at least in the short term.

"We'll do this just like last time," I said. "No shortcuts. And I need to see you every day to administer the CIWA scale, at least for the first week."

"You got it," he said.

I knew his odds of sustaining sobriety were poor. Of course, they were poor. He didn't have support. I was one of few cheerleaders urging him on, telling him he could do it, that things would be different this time.

Even under perfect conditions, his chance of lasting recovery wasn't great. Although estimates vary considerably, some studies show

40 percent of people who start AA drop out during the first year. Less than half the people who complete formal treatment or AA are sober eight years later. For those who don't attend a twelve-step program like AA or another post-detox aftercare program, only about a quarter will be abstinent from alcohol and drugs after one year.[1]

But we'd keep trying.

We would repeat the same cycle as before. Librium, the CIWA scale, daily visits, then every other day. He would see the counselor. He probably wouldn't go to AA. But we would get him detoxed, get him sober. I would be a nervous wreck for a couple of weeks, but I thought we could do it.

e⁓

I wasn't the only one with a difficult case. Terri's clinic session wasn't going so well either. Mrs. Davila, one of her long-standing and much-loved patients, had come in for her diabetes and cholesterol follow-up visit. Afterward, Terri had seen Mrs. Davila's nineteen-year-old granddaughter.

"She's pregnant," Terri said with a defeated sigh.

"Is she the one—?" I started to ask.

"Yes, Rosalia. She's the one who came in. . . . God, it seems like just a few weeks ago."

As Terri recalled, Rosalia had forgotten the required forms to qualify for free contraception. Terri had still written a prescription for birth control pills, but without funding, Rosalia hadn't picked them up.

"She's devastated," Terri said. "She says the father has just been deported."

"Oh my God. *Why* do we have to make it so hard for our patients to get birth control?" I asked. I didn't need to say it. We all agreed that contraception should be accessible and free for anyone who needed it.

While we gave out condoms regularly in the clinic, patients had to apply for special funds to cover the cost of birth control pills or Depo-Provera shots. They had to bring in paperwork, probably proof of residency, proof of (low) income—I don't even know. And we didn't have easy access to the most reliable methods: intrauterine devices and implants. Looking back, I wish I'd found a way to remove the obstacles, to provide same-day access to each woman's contraceptive of choice.

Barriers to birth control didn't make sense to me. They were short-sighted and didn't benefit anyone. Providing free, accessible contraception was both compassionate and economical. But most Texas legislators weren't known for their vision or basic math skills. Around the time of Rosalia's visit, Texas's teen birth rate was the fifth highest among all states in the country, yet schools weren't required to teach sex education. Other contributing factors included poverty, lack of health insurance, and high rates of school dropout.[2] Although rates have continued to decline over the last decade, Texas still ranks among the top-ten states for teen births.[3]

Those who needed care the most had the least access. Always. Andy couldn't access a safe detox program with the intensive post-detox support that might help him be successful. Rosalia couldn't get birth control, and now it was too late. So much suffering, *preventable* suffering, compounded thousands, even millions of times.

c⁀

Faith was waiting. I was running late, and as I entered the room, I braced myself for a litany of problems. But looking at her, I could tell something was different. She wasn't coughing; she was smiling. She had lost weight. A lot of weight.

"Sixty-five pounds!" she said as I shook her hand and sat down with my laptop to start recording her history in the EMR. I glanced at her vital signs. She was right. She had lost *sixty-five* pounds in just three months. Her blood pressure, blood sugar, and oxygen saturation were all within normal limits.

I looked at her again in astonishment. So much weight loss so fast was usually a cause for concern, but Faith looked healthier than I'd ever seen her. "That's amazing!" I said. "How did you do it?"

"Well, my asthma has been better, and they reduced my steroid dose at the asthma clinic," she said. "I've also been watching my diet— cutting out soda, eating more vegetables, like you said. I knew you'd be happy."

I couldn't believe it. For years, I'd watched her struggle, stuck in a vicious cycle of asthma requiring steroids causing weight gain and worsening health. Maybe she had broken free.

"That's amazing!" I repeated. "And I'm so glad you went to the asthma clinic. It looks like you saw the new counselor, too—I see her note here in the EMR."

"I'm trying, Dr. Doggett," she said. "My mood is better. The leg pain, too. It seems everything kind of goes together."

"You're not just trying. You're making really good progress. Way to go!"

As I refilled a couple of her medicines and typed my plan into her chart, I rejoiced in her progress. Medicine is so much more than mem-orizing drug names and recognizing patterns of symptoms. It's about relationships. I was part social worker, soothsayer, detective, cheer-leader. And my patients—Mauricio, Adriana, CJ, and Andy—each needed a different approach. Carlos needed three dollars and a reminder that his life meant something. Amber needed someone to listen and help her understand and treat a difficult diagnosis. At the core of it all was connection, establishing trust, forging an alliance.

Medicine is a team sport. While having smart and competent nurses and medical assistants is critical, the patient is always the most important team member. Ironically, it's because an individual's participation is so important and unpredictable that we need strong and compassionate systems to back them up. A safety net that's reliable, strong, without gaping holes, should be there to catch them. And we need to tailor an approach to care that fits each person's unique situation. Yet even in a flawed system, some patients, like Faith, would surprise me with their resilience. I knew such significant progress couldn't be expected with every patient and every visit, but hers was one victory I would celebrate.

CHAPTER 28

A Little Bird

March 2012

At each stage of my children's development—at least during the first few years—I was convinced with each passing month that we must have reached the Most Difficult Age. Occasionally, I realized that I was wrong. When Cathy's daughter, my eighteen-month-old niece, came for a playdate, I struggled to eliminate choking hazards, find a suitable snack, and mitigate the dangers of stairs and our enthusiastic dog, Clover. Adorable as she was, I was exhausted and relieved when Cathy came to pick her up after two hours. And I was reminded of the progress we'd made: Ella and Clara could stay alone in a room without extreme risk of injury or destruction. We could *talk* to each other. We were done with diapers!

But each age brought its own challenges, and the stubbornness and fury of four-year-old Clara convinced me with a renewed certainty that, like summiting a mountain on a long hike, we had reached the peak—the peak level of frustration, that is.

One typical morning, Clara fought for permission to eat breakfast in front of the TV so that she could watch *Curious George.* Then she wanted strawberries in her granola, not the peaches I had cut up. Every time she found something unsatisfactory, she would shout "No!" and demand something else. As we rushed to get ready, Clara wanted her butterfly tennis shoes, but they were lost. She did not want boots or flip-flops, and I ultimately convinced her to wear the tennis shoes with laces, though I knew the laces would come untied and flop around all day. We then had the usual battle to brush her hair: I chased and tackled Clara. As I touched her head with the brush, she screamed as if I was ripping out her fingernails.

But as we settled into the car at last, I glanced back at Ella. While I was preoccupied with her sister, Ella had independently combed her hair and put it into a ponytail. She was wearing appropriate clothes—jeans and a child-sized MIT (Don's alma mater) T-shirt—for school. She had loaded books into her backpack, filled her water bottle, and brushed her teeth.

"Thanks for getting ready so nicely, Ella," I said. "I think you're acting like a seven-year-old. Only one more week until your birthday, right?"

"Six days," Ella said.

"Six days. Right."

I remembered the night before when, after a disagreement about how many books she could get at the school book fair, Ella had gone to her room, written me a note of apology, and then come downstairs to say she was sorry and give me a hug. No knocking over bookshelves, no kicking or crying. Perhaps this child, who was only four when I was diagnosed with MS, was going to be okay, despite my weird disease. Those times that I was too dizzy to build a fort, or when I flipped out over a broken camera or a messy room . . . they hadn't ruined her life. I was imperfect. And she was going to be just fine anyway. Maybe—dare I hope?—she would be even more thoughtful, more compassionate because of my illness. At least now, thanks to Ella, I was catching a glimpse of the exit to the Waiting Place.

Someday, Clara would be seven, too. And if my dizziness continued to abate, I might even have the patience to guide her through the rest of childhood and beyond.

Ella's and Clara's birthday parties were often at our house with homemade cakes that always tasted much better than they looked. But Ella's celebration this year was a little more creative: an ice-skating party. Ever since Aunt Cathy had taken her skating at age four, Ella had been hooked. That fall, Ella had convinced me to sign her up for classes, and now she was, well, *good* at ice skating. She could glide, turn, and skate backward. She looked confident and graceful on the ice. I was awestruck watching her.

A few days before Ella's birthday, I dropped off Clara with my mom and headed with Ella toward the ice rink.

"We're going to get your birthday present," I told Ella.

"Where are we going?" she asked.

"You'll find out soon," I said.

Ella squirmed in the back seat, excited and impatient. "What's the present?" she asked more than once.

"You'll find out in just a few minutes," I replied, smiling at my own cleverness.

I had told Ella that she was too young for ice skates many times. Her feet were growing too fast; we needed to wait until she was older.

"But Mom, I need to get better skates. The rental ones are really bad," Ella would say.

"I understand. But new skates are expensive. Plus, I need to know that you're really going to stick with this, that you're not going to get tired of it." Now I was confident that my deceit was justified—and that Ella wouldn't quit anytime soon.

When we got to the ice-skating rink, Ella still wasn't sure what was going on.

"Am I getting a private lesson?" she asked.

"You'll find out soon," I repeated. "This way." I led her to the pro shop behind the rental skate counter. The small shop was crammed with ice skating clothing, blade guards, ice hockey sticks. We were met by a young skating instructor who wished Ella happy birthday and asked to measure her feet. Ella looked at me with bewildered delight as she realized she was getting her own pair of snow-white ice skates.

Ella's birthday party wasn't perfect. Many of the girls showed up in short-sleeved T-shirts and complained about the cold. Several had never skated before, and they stumbled around the ice, teeth chattering and wearing the extra adult-sized jackets I had thrown in the car at the last minute.

But Ella was elated. My parents and Cathy gathered at the rink with their well wishes and to watch her. She glided on her beautiful new skates with self-assurance, helping her friends who needed a hand to steady them on the ice. She wasn't a show-off, more like a little bird who had learned to fly and knew this was exactly what she was meant to do.

I ran with Jess the next morning, circling the lake together on the three-mile loop trail. We admired the bluebonnets—the state flower of Texas—and other wildflowers that seemed to have sprouted overnight.

"So how was the party?" she asked as we settled into our usual trot.

"Great. We had a few things go wrong, but it was still great," I said. "You know, I think my kid has found her calling."

"I'm so glad," she said.

"It may not last. I'm sure it'll change, but it's great to see her excitement, her passion."

Passion. Indeed, that was what I wanted for my kids—for them to find something that brought them joy, that motivated them to learn and work . . . to work hard.

But what about me? As we ran, I thought about my own interests. I could rattle off my goals: be a good doctor, a good mom, meet productivity targets at the clinic. I was on autopilot. Those were supposed to be my goals, so they were. But what was my passion? Traveling? Writing? Running? I hadn't thought about it in a long time. I was so focused on my kids and the clinic. Now that the kids were getting older and my MS was more manageable, maybe I could reconsider. Did I want to keep seeing patients? Did I want to think about new ways to promote health? Maybe I had learned from my MS experience and should share it in some way. Perhaps I could stray off my preplanned path—intentionally this time.

When we got near the bridge to take us back to our cars, I hesitated. "Should we try four miles today? I know we always do three. What do you think?"

"Sure. I've got time," Jess said.

"Let's go for it."

Ella didn't want to go to school the Monday after her birthday party.

"I don't want to go to work either," I said, imagining the new crisis that would be waiting. I wondered if I should, in fact, be honest about my hesitation. I wanted to model "find a job you love where you can make a difference." But I decided that acknowledging the highs and lows and showing persistence in the face of challenge was the more important lessons.

"I would rather be with you, but I have some patients who need my help," I said.

"I know," she said.

I continued, "You know, you may feel a little sad now, but I think that's a sign that you had a pretty great birthday. Sometimes when something is really good, you want to keep hanging on to it. And even though we may be sad today, I'm still so glad you had a wonderful birthday—and now you have a wonderful memory. You get to keep that memory."

Ella nodded. "When can we go back?"

"You have your skating lesson on Wednesday, and maybe we can go back to the rink just for fun this weekend. Would you like that?"

"I can wear my new skates!"

"Yes!" I smiled with her.

I paused as I picked up a small square of black paper lying on the kitchen counter. Ella had used a wooden stick to scratch away some of the black surface, revealing a rainbow of colors underneath. She had drawn a butterfly with a smiling face.

"I made that in art," Ella said. "I like the colors."

The colors were more vibrant because of the contrast with the black. I scratched the corner slightly with a fingernail. More colors jumped out.

It was like MS. That initial darkness had seemed so permanent. But now, when I could scratch through to the colors—my dizzy-free days, my adventures and accomplishments—they were more spectacular than ever.

"It's beautiful," I said, kissing her forehead. Then I grabbed my workbag to head to the clinic.

CHAPTER 29:
It's Happening

March 2012

My new patient, Lajuana, had breast cancer. The huge mass in her left breast felt like a jagged golf ball. Her overlying skin was thick and dark. Known as *peau d'orange*, the French term for "orange peel," the skin changes indicated a more advanced malignancy.

I tried to stay calm to cover my surprise at the size of the tumor. *Deep breath.* "I'm so glad you're here," I said. "I am concerned. . . . I know you are, too."

She nodded, sitting up on the table after I finished my exam. She clutched her paper gown in front with one hand and adjusted her red-framed glasses with the other.

She had first noticed the lump over a year ago.

"I knew it might be cancer, but I didn't have any insurance. I guess I just hoped it would go away," she said.

Lajuana finally had gone to Planned Parenthood the day before. They had ordered a mammogram and, knowing it would be abnormal, referred her to us. Our clinic had special grant funding to get a confirmatory biopsy and connect her with a breast specialist for further treatment. She was here to discuss her next steps.

"When was the last time you saw a doctor?" I asked.

"I don't know," she said, shifting a little in her seat. "It's been a while."

I was frustrated with her for waiting, but I understood. Delaying care is all too common, even among people with insurance—and it's gotten worse. A Gallup poll conducted in late 2022 showed that 38 percent of Americans reported that they or a family member had put off medical treatment in the last year because of the cost—a 12 percent increase over the previous year. People with low incomes and women are more likely to postpone care than other groups. Twenty-seven percent of survey respondents said that the delayed medical treatment was for a somewhat or very serious condition.[1] With Lajuana, I didn't know whether to hug or scold her.

"I'm a single mom. I used to have a good job, but my company downsized, and I got cut, so I lost my insurance," she said, perhaps sensing my need for an explanation. "My older daughter was diagnosed with ADHD, and she's had a really hard time in school. She kept getting expelled before we got her on the right medicines. I've just been preoccupied, I guess."

"Yeah, I get it. You've had a lot going on . . . but you did the right thing to come in, and now we can deal with it," I said. "I'll do my best to get you into the breast clinic as soon as possible."

I left the room to call again for the mammogram report, which still hadn't arrived on our fax machine. It was a typical worst-case scenario about which doctors commiserate at conferences. Her appointment was at the end of the day on a Friday afternoon. The mammogram had been done, and I was able to call the radiology center for a verbal report: Category Five, consistent with cancer. But I couldn't get a hard copy of the mammogram report in time to make the referral to the breast specialist, who wouldn't give her an appointment without having the report in hand. I worried that she wouldn't follow up without prompting and was afraid to let her leave the clinic without a future appointment to see the specialist.

I pleaded my case to the breast clinic receptionist. "Look, I know you all don't usually schedule appointments for patients without the mammogram report, but I have a verbal from radiology. This is a Category Five, and this lady's tumor is enormous. Can you please make an exception?"

The receptionist was annoyed with my urgency. "Our policy is that we can't make appointments for patients until the doctor here has reviewed the mammogram report," she said.

"Well, can I please talk to the doctor?" If I could only get the breast surgeon on the phone, perhaps they might relent. We could have that secret doctor-to-doctor handshake, and my patient could leave with a Monday morning appointment.

"All of our doctors are gone for the day," I was told. "The next available appointment isn't for two weeks anyway."

Of course. I was reminded of an image from a recent dream: my car trapped in a parking lot, blocked on all sides, and unable to move. It was Friday at 3:58 PM, two minutes before the breast clinic was due to close. My patient had waited a year to seek care. Another two weeks of waiting probably wouldn't make a difference. On the other hand, she was here now. She was suddenly motivated to get help, and I didn't want to miss an opportunity. I wasn't giving up, but I realized this person at the breast clinic was going to continue to stand in the way.

"Thanks," I said. "We'll call back on Monday." I hung up, thinking about my next steps. I had just lied to the receptionist. *Hell, if I'm going to wait until Monday.* And when the mammogram report finally arrived at 4:20 PM, confirming her Category Five status, I called the hospital operator and asked for the doctor on call for breast surgery. It worked. Five minutes later, the surgeon called back. I explained the situation, and she agreed to overbook an appointment for Lajuana, opening an extra slot on the schedule that was already full, on Monday. A small, hard-won success.

Earlier that week, I'd gone to a meeting to discuss productivity goals for the various community clinics. About thirty or forty doctors and other health care providers gathered in a crowded conference room adjacent to the children's hospital where Don worked. Together we watched the lead administrator share a PowerPoint presentation about what a tremendous disappointment we were. She didn't use those words, of course, but she showed slide after slide demonstrating that, month after month, we were failing to see the expected numbers of patients. Nearly all the clinics were well below the mark. In fact, over 80 percent of the doctors and nurse practitioners weren't meeting their productivity goals.

"Are we supposed to be surprised?" I whispered to the doctor seated next to me. "Their expectations are totally unrealistic."

She nodded in agreement.

The lead administrator pointed to a graph that looked to me like the financial tables of a company about to go bust. "Even though most people aren't meeting the goals, we know it's quite possible," she said.

Yeah, I thought. *I could meet their productivity goals if I never actually talked to a patient. If I didn't review the chart ahead of time. If I rushed in the room, skipped the medical history, and wrote a prescription for whatever the chief complaint happened to be. If I didn't care about creating trusting relationships or quality care.*

"We have at least one or two providers in each specialty area who are able to meet and, in some cases, surpass the productivity goals," she continued. "We need to get everyone up to that same standard."

That's it. She is delusional. I raised my hand.

"With all due respect, I disagree that the productivity goals are reasonable. Not all doctors are the same," I said. I didn't want to imply that other doctors were cutting corners. Some absolutely were capable of doing more in less time, but most of us couldn't do a good job and meet productivity expectations. I continued, "You know, some people can run a six-minute mile. I run every day, but I will never be able to run a six-minute mile."

The administrator stared at me. Surely, she could see the brilliance of my analogy. She let me go on.

"None of the medical providers at my clinic can meet the productivity goals. We can't do it with our existing patient population. Our patients are an important part of the team, but they are inefficient with inefficient problems."

I half expected the other doctors in the room to stand up and cheer, lifting me to their shoulders and singing, "For she's a jolly good fellow." But no one said anything.

The administrator smiled and mumbled something like "We have reason to believe these goals can be met." Then, louder, "Next slide!"

I wanted to drag the numbskull administrators into the exam room to see Lajuana. How could I counsel an uninsured woman about her breast cancer and arrange an urgent specialty clinic appointment in fifteen minutes? And what about my other patients? How could I hurry an obese nine-year-old with prediabetes, who had gained another ten pounds in the weeks since her older sister—her role model and best friend—had run away? Could they come tell me which problem to ignore for the patient who showed up complaining of severe headaches, anxiety, and abdominal pain?

"See! This can't be done quickly!" I would say. "Are you really telling me I should spend only ten or fifteen minutes with these patients so I can meet your productivity goals? And we're supposed to use that terrible EMR to do it? Don't even get me started on that."

I feel certain my own MS would have been missed had I been uninsured, unable to advocate for myself, and crammed into a fifteen-minute appointment slot. Even if the doctor had taken the time to ask questions, vague dizziness with vague visual complaints and a normal exam would have been dismissed as anxiety, stress, a viral infection. If my symptoms had persisted, I might have been started on a medicine for depression before the doctor had to rush out of the room, without a second thought, to tend to her next patient.

Among those who receive an MS diagnosis, people with low incomes don't do as well as their more affluent counterparts. They are more likely to have vision loss, anxiety, depression, and other comorbid medical conditions.[2] It's no wonder. Many, I'm sure, are stuck receiving care at clinics struggling to increase "patient volume" and just stay afloat.

Deep listening skills, medical curiosity, empathy, and persistence are traits common to the best doctors, but they are discouraged and devalued in a system obsessed with efficiency and productivity numbers. The consequences are poor documentation, rushed visits, a burned-out workforce, and—absolutely—missed diagnoses and sub-optimal care.

c⁓

Despite my cynicism about the administration's expectations, I came up with a plan. In addition to the new exam rooms and improved front office space created by the recent remodel, I restructured our schedules and hired a new doctor. Smart and kind, Dr. Hanser quickly built a panel of devoted patients with complex health problems. I was delighted to have her support and camaraderie in the clinic.

Over the next few months, I tracked and scrutinized our schedules the way Wall Street executives must monitor the stock market. Maybe Terri could add one more appointment on Wednesday afternoons. Our part-time endocrinologist could see one more patient on Tuesdays. Maybe I could fit in one more before lunch on Fridays. We modified our intake process. We adjusted our no-show policy and made appointment reminder calls to reduce the numbers of patients who failed to show up for their visits. Many of our sister clinics eliminated the physicians' administrative time. I refused to follow suit, arguing that admin time was essential to allow us to review labs and specialty consult notes, refill prescriptions, and prepare for upcoming clinic sessions. But I felt compelled to make every second count. The pressure to meet our numbers goals was greater than ever, as was my resentment about those goals. Medicine wasn't a numbers game. I hadn't become a doctor to meet productivity goals. I wanted to help people.

Seeing Mrs. Reyes reminded me of that. An elderly woman originally from a village near Mexico City, she stood up to embrace me and kiss my cheek when I walked into the exam room. She was always accompanied by one of her eleven children, all grown, and sometimes a grandchild or two. That day, one of her daughters sat next to her, and she nodded and smiled as I entered.

Like many of my patients, Mrs. Reyes had high blood pressure, but I had also diagnosed her with chronic obstructive pulmonary disease (COPD). During one of our first visits together, she had reported a long-standing cough and occasional wheezing, and I had ordered pulmonary function testing—an evaluation to see how the lungs are working. The results showed an obstructive lung disease that did not respond to bronchodilator therapy. In other words, she had a classic pattern for COPD, seen most often in smokers.

"I know you don't smoke now, but did you ever smoke?" I'd asked in Spanish.

"Only when I was pregnant," she responded. "They said it would be good for the baby."

"They?" This was a new one.

"Yes, the doctors."

"Hmm . . . Okay, and you've had how many pregnancies—eleven?" I asked.

"No, thirteen pregnancies. I lost two," she said.

Smoking throughout thirteen pregnancies and living near a large, polluted city for most of her life would explain the COPD. I managed to get her started on a newer medication through the drug company's free patient assistance program. She had been doing well.

"*Doctora Lisa,*" she now said to me as I settled on my stool. "I'm so happy to see you again."

"I'm happy to see you, too. It's been a while." I scanned through her chart, noting she'd missed her last appointment.

"She went to Mexico," her daughter said. "Her sister died, and she had to go back for about six months."

"Oh, I'm sorry to hear that," I said. "Did you see any doctors in Mexico?"

"No, she wanted to wait to see you," her daughter said.

"Only you are my doctor," Mrs. Reyes said, smiling at me.

I felt flattered . . . and maybe a little suffocated. But I smiled back at her and squeezed her outstretched hand.

After refilling her medications and discussing some ways to improve her diet, I picked up my laptop and headed for the door. Mrs. Reyes intercepted to hug me.

"I'm so glad you're my doctor," she said, and then in English, "I love you."

I hugged her back, remembering how uncomfortable I used to feel when a patient said that to me. I used to feel confused about how to respond and would say something like "You're so sweet." But then I thought, *Why not say I love these patients? They drive me crazy and stress me out, but I care about them deeply.* I decided that I wasn't jeopardizing our doctor-patient relationship or being unprofessional to say I loved them back. Love shouldn't be restricted to a select few. The more, the better.

"I love you, too," I said.

c⁓

Elizabeth and I gathered with Kim in front of her computer. None of us could believe it. Now that Dr. Hanser was on our team, Terri was working full-time, and the rest of us were adding patients where we could, we had met our productivity target for the second month in a row. It also helped that we finally had the medical assistants and front desk staff we needed. The last month, when we had achieved our goal for the first time, had been exciting. I had thought it could be a fluke. But two months in a row? That was something!

"I'm counting six visits over our target. That doesn't even include the counselor's appointments," Kim said. "How many did you get, Elizabeth?"

"I counted twenty-two above the goal. I think the discrepancy is because some of the encounter forms haven't been fully processed," Elizabeth said.

"So, we are really meeting our goal?" I asked, giddy with the realization. "I mean, even if we go by Kim's numbers, we're there!"

"I think so," Elizabeth said. "I've counted three times."

"Oh my God! We have been trying to do this for so long!" I said. We were working hard. We were *not* finishing our notes by 5:00 PM every day, and I had negotiated more reasonable numbers for our clinic than the original goal. But I still felt like we had just won the Olympics.

Don and I had an inside joke that was also a coping technique: During some of our worst moments, when the smoke alarm was screeching because our dinner was burned or the kids were fighting or screaming, we would look at each other and say with wry irony, "It's happening." The expression was supposed to convey the sentiment that all our wishes and fantasies were coming true. But we used it, instead, with extreme sarcasm, when those hopes and dreams were flailing on the ground in tears. We made fun of our past naïve optimism—about parenting, about our future—with that expression.

I didn't say it now, but the thought, *It's happening,* broadened my smile because, for once, it seemed real.

Sara Maria interrupted our little celebration. "Dr. Doggett, you've got another patient in room six."

"Okay, one second," I said. I smiled again at Kim and Elizabeth. "Thanks, y'all. This has been a big team effort. I guess I better go make sure we keep our numbers up." I headed to the exam room.

CHAPTER 30:

A Pebble in My Shoe

June 2013

One evening, on the way home from her ice-skating lesson, Ella surprised me with an odd revelation. "The end of the words looks blurry when I read," she said. "So, I'm not reading as much now."

"What do you mean—'the end of the words'?'" I asked. "Only part of the words looks blurry?"

"You don't understand," Ella said. She was seated behind me, and I glanced at her in the rearview mirror. She was staring out the window, scowling.

"I want to understand. Can you help me? You said the end of the words look blurry—like the last few letters?"

"You don't understand," Ella repeated.

I didn't. I tried to coax her to tell me more, but she insisted I didn't and couldn't understand, so I let it drop. But the worry stayed with me, nagging like a pebble in my shoe.

My first MS symptoms, before the dizziness, the random numbness, and taste changes—before I really suspected Something Bad—had been visual changes. I never received a solid explanation for those initial symptoms, but I knew that many people with MS experienced visual abnormalities, often as the first indication of disease. Optic neuritis, a rare condition caused by inflammation of the optic nerve, is relatively common in MS. It can cause changes in color perception, pain that is usually worse with eye movement, and even blindness. MS lesions along the neurologic pathways that control eye movements can cause visual changes as well. My vision was never blurry, but cloudy in the months leading up to my diagnosis. It was hard to explain what that meant, in the same way that it was hard to explain what my dizziness felt like. But it did make reading hard sometimes, and it was intermittent and difficult to characterize.

That evening, after Ella was asleep, I mentioned it to Don.

"She told me the same thing," he said. "She wouldn't cooperate when I tried to get her to read a couple pages of *Harry Potter* tonight. She said something like she couldn't see the ends of the sentences."

Don and I knew better than to press Ella on an unpleasant topic. "Pick your battles" was our shared mantra. Her symptoms didn't make sense. They didn't fit any diagnosis, even pediatric MS. We told each other that "it's probably nothing."

Still, I couldn't just dismiss it. Don and I agreed to watch for anything new and to get help if she continued to complain.

The next day, I made a point to check Ella's eyesight. I didn't have a chart with the big E like we had at the clinic, but I used a book and tried to test both near and far vision.

Ella didn't want to be tested, and she would read seven or eight letters, and then say she couldn't read any more because it was blurry.

I made her try on my glasses, to see if maybe that would improve her vision. I knew it was silly. She would never have the same prescription, but I just wanted a clue about what was going on.

"Hello, Professor Ella." I laughed. "You look so old in my glasses. Do you teach chemistry or are you a professor of ice skating?"

"I don't know what you're talking about," Ella said, taking off the glasses, embarrassed.

"Wait, try them again," I said.

She frowned but put the glasses on.

"I know it's weird, but Ella, do you think you can see any better with them?" I asked.

"I think so," she said, but when I tried to retest her vision with the glasses on, she either couldn't see or wasn't trying. I couldn't tell. The test was officially inconclusive.

"Is it hard for you to see the board at school?" I asked her.

"No . . . I don't know. We don't use the board very much," she replied. "You don't understand. It's not such a big deal, Mom."

Ella's lifetime odds of getting MS were about one in twenty-five, according to Dr. Reynard. That was much higher than the general population, though still favorable for not getting it. In addition, pediatric MS is rare, accounting for only about 5 percent of cases. But by the third or fourth day of symptoms, when Ella still refused to read, mentioning her blurry vision again to her dad, Don started to panic.

Don's anxiety took the shape of irritability. Any question or request, from the kids or me, was met with a reluctant sigh and an exasperated "What now?" Saturday afternoon, after Don finished a morning of work, I wanted to send him—and his negativity—back to the hospital.

"Why are you so grumpy?" I asked more than once.

"I'm not!" he insisted.

I didn't make the connection to Ella until after the kids were in bed that evening.

"I talked with the pediatric ophthalmologist today," Don said, when at last we were alone. "I ran into her at the hospital this morning, and I told her about Ella's symptoms. She can see her next week."

"Okay, well that sounds reasonable. What did she say?"

"She said lots of kids have visual changes at Ella's age. She probably just needs glasses," he answered.

"Alright, so that's okay, right? Not a big deal," I said. "Did that help you feel better?"

"Well at first, yeah, but then Ella mentioned it again this afternoon." He sighed. "I just can't stand the thought of her having MS, too."

I was caught between Don's paranoia and my own concerns. On a gut level, I was terrified. The idea that my kid could have MS was so much worse than having it myself. And I couldn't escape that feeling, however irrational, that it would somehow be my fault. While MS wasn't contagious or even inherited in a blue eyes/brown eyes sort of way, Ella's odds were increased because of me.

On the other hand, Don was shouldering enough worry for both of us. By that point, we didn't know if Ella was even serious about her symptoms. Her descriptions were vague, and we had reacted with such heightened concern that perhaps we had encouraged her to exaggerate and perseverate. I'd also learned with MS that our ability to make predictions was limited. Uncertainty created anxiety, but it also offered hope. And we could be resilient, no matter what.

"We're too biased to sort this out," I said to Don. "I think she's going to be okay, but let's take her to the eye doctor and get someone who isn't her parent to weigh in." It should have been a no-brainer.

A few days later, Don called from the parking lot outside the ice-skating rink. They had just seen the eye doctor. He and Ella were sitting in his car, and I could hear Ella crying in the background.

"It's normal. The exam, the vision tests—all normal. She doesn't even need glasses," he said, his voice infused with familiar anxiety. "We discussed doing an MRI. The ophthalmologist ordered it, but she doesn't think Ella needs it. She says she sees this pattern—kids complaining of visual changes—all the time, and it's not a concern."

"Okay. What's going on? Why is Ella crying?"

"She doesn't want to get an MRI, and now she is refusing to go to her ice-skating class."

Don was near tears himself. The doctor's words should have been reassuring, but they only fueled Don's obsessive fear. He wanted an explanation for Ella's complaints, and a normal exam didn't provide one. I could hardly blame him. When I had visual changes, before my MS diagnosis, I was examined by a general ophthalmologist and then a retina specialist, who said I had dry eyes. No one had suspected MS. Even I didn't connect the dots until several weeks after my MRI and spinal tap. When I realized that my MS had been missed by these doctors, I wanted to send them my MRI report with the white spots. I would attach a note: "'Dry eyes,' huh?"

MS had shown Don and me that our imagined shield, which we once assumed protected us from calamity, was a mirage. We had fortified that shield. Seat belts, smoke alarms, life jackets, bike helmets— we embraced them all. If I heard thunder on a run, I turned around. We kept a fire extinguisher by the fireplace. We followed dietary guidelines—five or more cups of fruits and veggies every day. We sweated through at least "150 minutes of moderate-intensity physical activity a week," per national exercise recommendations. And still, we were vulnerable. Even worse, our kids were vulnerable. We could do everything right and still end up with dizziness and cloudy vision and white spots.

Now Don was sitting there with our sobbing child, thinking of all the Somethings Bad. A brain tumor or MS—they were unlikely, but still possible. He didn't ask for my advice, but I could tell he needed it. And if Ella was refusing to ice skate, which she loved, she was unhinged as well.

"I'm coming out there," I said. "I just saw my last patient, and I can finish my notes later. I'll be there in about fifteen minutes."

As I drove to the ice rink parking lot, I concocted a plan. First, I needed to get over the fact that Ella was missing her ice-skating class that day. Her lessons were expensive, and I hated for her to skip one. Skating also was rejuvenating for her, like restorative yoga for me. If she could skate, she would feel better. But I needed to let it go.

Second, I needed to support Don. As frustrated as I was with his irrationality and recent bad mood, I knew he was struggling and scared because of his love for our daughter. And what if he was right? What if Ella had Something Bad? It was too much to think about. The situation was triggering flashbacks to my diagnosis for both of us. That time, so riddled with uncertainty and fear, had highlighted our fragility. Don and I were on the same team. I needed to remember that.

Finally, I needed to decide whether to get the MRI for Ella. Would we be getting a medically indicated test or treating our own anxiety? I wasn't sure.

I located Don's car in the parking lot, pulled up next to it, and climbed in. I tried to hug Ella in the back seat, but she pushed me away and began crying again. I settled in the front seat next to Don and took his hand.

"Does the ophthalmologist feel like there is any real reason to get the MRI?" I asked.

"Not really. I was the one pushing for it. I think she didn't want to upset me since I'm a colleague. She said that it's common for kids to have this. I just can't—" his voice broke. I squeezed his hand and leaned over to hug him.

"It's going to be okay," I said. "Let's get out of this hot parking lot and go talk somewhere."

I suggested a coffee shop nearby, and Don drove us there, glancing at Ella through the rearview mirror every few seconds.

"She's going to be fine," I said again, trying to reassure him, though Ella was in the car with us, and I didn't want to keep talking about her like she wasn't there. His mind was spinning, caught up in possibilities, far-fetched though they might be. I recalled the time that Don thought Clara's fever and fussiness could be meningitis. Arguing that she just had a cold, I had to stop him from rushing her to the ER at 2:00 AM. His work as a hospital-based pediatrician brought him in contact with the sickest kids in the city every day. He saw kids with every manner of Something Bad diseases—rare cancers, autoimmune conditions, infections, random accidents. His increased concern that our kids could have a serious illness when they reported symptoms wasn't surprising. Though he was a master diagnostician, his judgment was clouded when our kids were concerned. My MS diagnosis had compounded his fear, his pessimistic tendencies.

I got drinks for all of us, and we sat down at a table in the coffee shop. Ella perked up with her strawberry smoothie. I patted her shoulder and looked at Don.

"Look, if we do the MRI, are we treating Ella or you?" I asked.

He didn't answer.

"An MRI has its own risks, even if they are small," I continued.

"I don't want an MRI," Ella said.

"I know, Ella. I don't blame you. We're just trying to make the best decision for you," I said. I looked again at Don, realizing we probably shouldn't have this conversation in front of Ella but feeling compelled to continue. "You can't be your own kid's doctor," I said. "I know that things can be missed. But I think we need to be glad Ella's eye exam was normal and follow the ophthalmologist's advice."

"I guess we can wait a few days," he said.

"We don't have to make a decision yet."

Ella's symptoms resolved, and no new symptoms developed. To this day we can't explain what happened. She didn't have MS. Or maybe she did, God forbid, and it would resurface later with new symptoms. But we needed to put our fears aside and be rational, realize it was unlikely. Don's conversation with a pediatric neurologist reassured us our kid was okay. Pediatric MS is uncommon, even with a family history. Odds were in favor of her staying healthy. Best news ever.

CHAPTER 31:

I Never Thought I'd Leave

June 2014

Hard to believe, but I was leaving my practice. Nearly two years had passed since we first met our productivity goals. More than four years had passed since my MS relapse, with no subsequent flares. But now, seven years after becoming the director of a tiny, unknown clinic in Central Austin, after building my dream team and caring for hundreds—no, thousands—of patients there, it was time to move on. I had picked out tile for the floors, hung paintings on the walls, and spent a good chunk of my life meeting people from all over the world, unraveling their stories, and trying, in some small way, to help. With some, like Faith, I felt a sense of progress, a tangible improvement in her health that we had accomplished as a team. With others, like Tiffany, I couldn't see that I'd made a bit of difference. And with many, I was left wondering what happened because they didn't come back. Maybe they had given up, moved somewhere else, found a new doctor, or even gotten private insurance. I would never know.

The decision to leave was both easy and agonizing. Productivity pressures and EMR challenges had continued to plague me. So-called leadership changes compromised my ability to operate the clinic effectively and care for my patients. During the time when I was considering a transition, I had cut back my hours at the clinic and taken a part-time position as medical director for a statewide program to support children with special needs and health concerns. I worked with a team of nurses and social workers across Texas to identify and assist families who needed help accessing care for their kids with asthma, autism, cerebral palsy, and other chronic conditions. I wanted to devote more time to that initiative, and I needed a break from clinical practice.

Still, I worried about my patients. Who else would fight to get them specialty care, to find low-cost medications? I was their confidante, their ally, their advocate. But I was giving myself too much credit. They would see other doctors—maybe better, smarter doctors. I wasn't the only person who could help. And after seven years, my shelf life was up. The idealized version of the good ol' family doc, who sees patients from cradle to grave, was almost extinct. New opportunities to learn and contribute awaited me. With feelings of both regret and relief, a sense of loss and hope, I would move on, and so would my patients.

My last patient visits before my departure included many of my regulars . . . and some unexpected reunions. Andy had disappeared for a long time, maybe a year or more. We had called to check on him, when he missed a follow-up appointment, but never connected. I hoped he was sober. Perhaps he had found private insurance coverage, maybe even a job, but I feared he was struggling somewhere, that he was drinking again. I was surprised to see his name on my schedule, a couple of weeks before I left. I wondered what could have prompted the visit, what it would be like. *Could he be better? Could we possibly have been successful at getting him to stop drinking? Dare I hope for a miracle?*

A woman was in the room with him when I opened the door. She was professionally dressed, with slacks and a button-down shirt. His wife—or ex-wife, at least. The one who checked on him during detox. The one who couldn't completely give up on him either. I was so glad to see her.

"I'm Carol," she said, shaking my hand. "I'm his . . . ex-wife. I'm . . . well, I brought Andy in today. I'm concerned." Her smile was strained. She was worn-out. We both turned to Andy.

"Hey," he said, looking up at me. He was slouched over in the chair. He was holding a cane.

"Oh Andy, I'm so glad to see you," I said, reaching out to grasp his hand. "I've thought of you so many times."

"I've thought of you, too," Andy said, his voice flat, tired. "I didn't want to disappoint you."

"He's been drinking," Carol said. "He stopped for several months after the last time he detoxed, but then he disappeared for a couple days."

"I couldn't stop. I just couldn't help it," he said.

"I kept checking on him—or trying to," Carol continued. "When I got in touch with him, he was pretty sick. He wouldn't come see you until now."

Andy looked ten years older. His hands trembled, and I couldn't tell if he was withdrawing, or it was something else. He told me he was in pain—back, legs, feet.

"He's pretty depressed," Carol said, "and his memory seems to be getting worse."

I conducted a brief exam. His heart and lungs sounded normal, and his abdominal exam was unremarkable, though I knew that didn't rule out liver problems. But, on his neurologic exam, Andy was shaky and slow, struggling with the finger-to-nose and heel-to-shin tests as well as tandem gait, indicating problems with coordination and balance. He also couldn't localize his pain to one area, and I didn't know what to suggest. Perhaps he had Parkinson's, but it would be hard to sort that out while he was still drinking heavily. I'd start with some basic labs and at least assess his liver function.

"Let's get you in to see the counselor," I said. "We have a new person, and I think you'll like her. She may have some ideas about how to get more help with your drinking. Then I'll see you back after you get those lab tests."

"Yeah, okay," he said.

He didn't ask to be detoxed. I didn't suggest it. He was too high risk at that point to try an outpatient regimen. Carol had a lead on a possible inpatient facility—something new that I had never heard of—and I offered to assist in any way I could.

Before he left, I took his hand again. "Hey—don't worry about disappointing me," I said. "Stopping drinking . . . it's really, really hard. If you can't do it . . . I'm still here for you. I wanna help."

But he never came back. He scheduled an appointment on his way out, but then he canceled or didn't show up. I never saw him again.

It was hard not to be disappointed in myself. I didn't blame myself exactly, but I wondered if I could have done more to find support for Andy after his detox. Maybe I should have pushed harder for AA or called to check on him more often. Maybe I should have reached out to Carol or someone else. Usually, I know my limits, and sometimes I push past them, stretching them like a bungee cord. Each patient has his own story, his own vices and victories. I search for each person's strengths and try to build on them. I use available resources and tools, and I search for more when I need them. Maybe going to AA and having better treatment would have made a difference. Maybe not. But I know Andy needed me to go out of my way, outside my comfort zone, and I did. I fought for him when no one else would . . . because no one else would. It wasn't enough to save him, but maybe he got a few more months of life as a result—a few more walks with his dogs, a few days or weeks to hope and dream about a future, even if it was not to be.

⇛

"I brought you a present," Mrs. Waller said when I entered the room for our last visit together. With her good hand, she reached into her purse, which hung from the arm of her wheelchair. She handed me a small box.

"Oh, that's very nice of you, truly . . . but it's unnecessary," I said.

"It's not much. Just one of my old things that I thought you'd like," she said. "I heard you're leaving, and I just wanted to thank you."

I opened the box and pulled out a garnet necklace. "I love it," I said, looking at her and smiling. I meant it. It was my style—vintage, unique, not fancy. I could have picked it out myself.

I always felt guilty accepting a gift from a patient, but I also knew from her smile and expectant expression that refusing the gift was not an option.

I put the necklace on and took her stiff hand in both of mine. "I'm glad to see you again. How are you feeling?"

"A little better, I think. Still some pain in my back," she said.

"I know. That's frustrating—hard to live with," I said. She was trying physical and occupational therapy again, at least to learn to transfer herself in and out of the wheelchair more independently. Her progress was slow. Most of her limitations were permanent and significant. We had succeeded in controlling her cholesterol and blood pressure, but I didn't feel like I had much else to offer.

"I just wish I could get back to walking. I'd like to teach, maybe high school," she said.

I didn't know what to say. She wasn't going to regain the abilities she'd lost. Not this long after her stroke. I think she knew, too, that she was wishing for the impossible.

"That would be wonderful," I said. "I think you'd be a great teacher."

I didn't want to shoot down her dreams. If she had asked me directly, I would have told her she would probably never walk again. I would have redirected her to focus on more realistic goals and everyday pleasures.

"Well, it may not happen, but you never know," she said.

"You never know," I repeated.

⁓

Faith came to say goodbye with a gift as well. She didn't have an appointment, but she dropped by with a mysterious object, awkward and wrapped in newspaper.

"I just wanted to say thank you," she said, handing me the package. "I'm really gonna miss you."

Faith. It was hard to say goodbye. As much as she had challenged me over the years, I had looked forward to her friendly greetings and admired her determination to power through with her asthma and chronic knee pain. She was always grateful, even when I had to send her back to the ER in the midst of a bad asthma exacerbation, even when I couldn't do much of anything to help.

I unwrapped the gift to reveal a mobile with colorful glass birds hanging from a metal spiral. Orange, red, and blue, the birds were cheerful and playful but still delicate. They would be perfect hanging outside the window of my office at home. I felt tears in my eyes.

"I love it," I said.

A month—and a vacation—after my last day at the clinic, I gathered with Kim, Sara Maria, Elizabeth, Terri, and all the others—about fifteen of us by that point—for a festive going-away party. Terri hosted us at her house, and I brought Clara with me for the Tex-Mex potluck and a dip in the pool. Everyone wore summer attire—flowery patterns, bold colors—as we sipped iced tea and wine on the deck.

"We're getting another EMR upgrade," Terri said. "I bet you're sorry to be missing out on that."

I laughed. "And are they telling you it's going to be a thousand times better? All the kinks are worked out, and it will make everyone's workflow so much better?"

"Yeah, I'm not that optimistic," Terri said. "We'll see."

Our potlucks were always epic, and this one was no different. We feasted on tacos, three different kinds of salad, guacamole, chips, and

queso. Sara Maria had ordered my favorite—an Italian cream cake—
for dessert.

"Faith's still doing well," Kim reported. "She wanted me to tell you,
'Hi.' Her husband has been in the hospital, but I think he's back home
now."

"I'm sorry to hear that. I know that's hard on her. Please tell her I
said 'Hi' back."

We caught up, reminisced, and laughed all evening.

"Remember when we had the mice?" someone asked.

"Oh my God. Yeah, and the Joint Commission was coming."

"Remember when the vaccine refrigerator broke?"

"Remember when it flooded in the back office?"

"Remember when we finally met our productivity goals?"

At one point, Clara dragged me into the pool for a silly, disjointed
game of Marco Polo, but I coaxed her out again for a group photo with
the suggestion that we should cut the cake.

Before we left, my clinic family presented me with a beautiful new
workbag and a gift certificate to continue my restorative yoga classes
(hopefully without the accompaniment of chain saws). I was humbled
and so grateful.

"You know me well," I said. "It's perfect."

I thought of all those evenings when I'd driven home, overwhelmed
with stress and self-doubt. I felt guilty to be abandoning the trenches,
taking a break from the chaos—maybe a permanent one. *Was I leaving too much undone, was I giving up too soon? So many of my patients
did not have happy endings. Did those seven years at the clinic really
amount to anything?* Now, as I swapped stories with my coworkers
(friends) and discussed future plans, my team was helping to convince
me that maybe I'd accomplished something.

I didn't want to leave that night, but I knew I would see nearly everyone again. We were forever connected through the months and years of shared struggles, working toward a common goal, accompanied by intense frustrations and occasional successes. Like old army buddies, we would keep in touch.

CHAPTER 32

This Is the Way It Is Right Now

September 2014

L eaving the clinic was necessary, but in doing so, I had pulled up an anchor. After investing so much in my work, I now needed to find a new direction, explore new opportunities. Ultimately, I caved to peer pressure, and I emerged better for it.

For years, two close doctor friends had sung the praises of meditation with an almost evangelical zeal.

"It changed my life," Kerry said more than once. "I'm more peaceful, calm, and intentional."

"It's a different way of seeing things," Marcie said. "A new way of being in a kinder relationship with yourself and with others."

It sounded a little woo-woo to me. But Marcie persisted. "You know, I even teach my patients. Mindfulness meditation allows you the ability to observe what's happening and not get so wrapped up in it."

I didn't get it. Sitting still—doing nothing, as I thought of it—just increased my anxiety. My mind became a beehive of sharp thoughts. I spent those moments planning the next ones, reviewing my task list, impatient to start working through it. Or I perseverated on my topsy-turvy career. Just a couple of months after my going-away party, I had jumped at the unexpected opportunity to serve as medical director at a clinic for immigrant families. My part-time medical director position had turned out to be too part-time, and I saw the new clinic as a chance to serve a vulnerable population, but without some of the bureaucratic strings of my last job. Still, I worried that the new clinic would soon swallow me whole. Was I up to the challenge?

I thought that meditation meant clearing my mind. And I couldn't clear my mind. Since my thoughts were so constant and intrusive, if I tried to meditate, surely I'd end up berating myself for my inability to do it right.

But like the catchy jingle of an advertisement on TV, the idea of meditation stayed with me.

I called my friend Marcie, my roommate and best friend from medical school, to find out more. As I listened to Marcie's update on her family medicine job and life in Seattle, I walked through the neighborhood with my dog, trying to spot the cats before Clover leaped at them. I loved catching up with my sweet friend. When she finished with her update, I broached a new topic.

"So, I wanted to ask you. This meditation that you do . . . if somebody was going to start, how would they do it?"

"Oh," she said, laughing. "Asking for a friend, are you?"

"You got me," I said. "I'm not for sure yet, but I'm thinking about trying it."

"That's great," she said, "and there are lots of ways to start—books, meditation apps. But I think the MBSR class is definitely worth considering."

"The what?"

"Yeah, there's a Mindfulness-Based Stress Reduction—MBSR—class you can take. It's usually once a week for eight weeks, and you learn the basics of meditation," she said. "I've taken it twice."

She went on to explain that mindfulness is a form of mediation that emphasizes awareness of the present moment. "You may think it's whack-a-doodle, but it's backed by scientific studies showing improvements in physical and emotional well-being in regular practitioners."

I'm a sucker for a scientific study, but I still wasn't ready to commit. *Eight weeks? I can't do it,* I thought. *I don't have time, I'm incapable of meditating, I can't sit still.*

Then I ran into another doctor friend. "I have a friend who is teaching a meditation class—Mindfulness-Based Stress Reduction," she said. "She is particularly interested in having some doctors participate."

Maybe the universe was trying to get my attention.

The class was close to my house, just once a week. Logistically, it could work. The sessions targeted stress, my nemesis. I certainly could use more tools to fight stress. Maybe my reasons not to take the class—too much going on, an endless to-do list, feeling pulled in too many directions—were the same reasons that I should do it. I could learn to slow down, to focus. Forever troubled by the fleeting nature of the present—the fact that every event, every action, is either past or future—I wondered if meditation might help me feel more grounded, more in-the-moment. I could be more present with my patients and with my kids. I could share what I learned with others.

I invited Don to join me. I worried that he would think it was too weird, too alternative. Or maybe we'd get a chatty teacher like the instructor from my ill-fated yoga class. Oh, I'd never hear the end of it. But his anxiety was triggered by my MS. Maybe meditation would help us both. To my relief, he agreed. He wanted to support me, and he was willing to give it a try.

The room was sparse, uncluttered. People were gathering in a circle in the middle of the room, some with yoga mats, others with cushions or blankets. I rolled out my gray mat on the wood floor and sat down.

"Welcome. I'm Geeta," said our instructor—an Indian woman a few years older than me, with curly, shoulder-length black hair. She had a warm smile, kind eyes. In fact, kindness emanated from her.

We sat on the floor in half chairs that had backs and seats but no legs.

"Thank you for joining our class," Geeta said, sitting down cross-legged, acknowledging each person with eye contact and a smile.

Geeta guided us through our first mindful meditation, lasting just a few minutes. "Bring your attention to your breath," she said. "Notice the inhale and the exhale. Feel your breath as your chest rises and falls."

I listened to her gentle voice. I didn't have to clear my head, just concentrate on my breath. *Easy enough. I can do that.*

Next, Geeta handed out raisins.

No incense or Tibetan gongs?

"Put it in your mouth," she instructed. "Notice the texture."

I felt the raisin's tiny furrows, its oval shape, turning it over in my mouth.

"Notice if there is any taste to the raisin yet, even before you chew or swallow it."

For five minutes, we each ate a single raisin. It was the most I have ever focused on a bite of food. I thought of adjectives to describe it, but then I realized I didn't have to. In fact, I didn't "have to" do anything.

Eating the raisin was an exercise, Geeta explained, to heighten our awareness of the present, where we spend all our time physically, but very little time mentally. Instead of noticing the present, I spent my time planning the future or reliving the past. I was missing out on many of my raisins.

Geeta answered my most pressing question during our first class before I could even ask.

"While meditating, thoughts will come to you," she said. "That's okay. You can regard them. Acknowledge them with kindness, without judgment. Then let them go."

I tried it. I sat and concentrated on my breath and Geeta's words during a longer meditation at our next session. When I caught myself rehashing the day, instead of reprimanding myself for failing to stick with the present moment, I thought, *Oh! I was just thinking about my day. Now I'm going to focus on my breath again. This is a mindful moment.*

These unusual date nights for Don and me, spent in silent meditation, followed by a group debriefing, became a fixture of our week. The class offered a welcome way to reconnect. Often, we were rushed, after busy days at work, to make it on time, but it was worth the effort.

"Don, grab the yoga mats," I'd shout, slipping on my shoes as I gave instructions—rapid-fire—to the sitter. "Pasta and broccoli—can you steam it? Maybe cut up an apple. Then baths. Ella may need help with homework. If you can get Clara down, that's awesome, but it's probably too much to hope for."

Sometimes we managed to arrive in time for dinner at Casa de Luz, the beautiful macrobiotic, vegan restaurant next door to our meditation meeting room. Don adjusted his hospital schedule so that he could attend each class, and on other nights, we would complete the exercises in our workbook together. I also added a six-minute morning meditation to my waking-up routine.

In class, we learned about different methods of meditation. Focusing on the breath was the most common and obvious form. But body scan, walking meditation, sound meditation, and mindful movement, or yoga, added variety to our practice.

"Take a moment now to check in with yourself," Geeta would say, as we started a group session. "If you notice discomfort, sit with it for a minute with kindness and curiosity. You may even invite it in for tea, like a houseguest. There is no need to judge or even try to change it. Just remind yourself that this is the way it is right now."

Camila was a thirty-five-year-old woman with chronic abdominal pain and depression. I saw her in the first few weeks at my new clinic and liked her immediately. We bonded over child-rearing challenges, and she told me about her new food truck business selling *arepas, empanadas,* and other Colombian meals and snacks.

"I can't wait to come pick up dinner at your truck," I said on our second visit. "I'm glad that's working out so far."

"Thanks," she said. "I'm glad, too, but I just . . . I don't know. I thought I'd feel better once it got going, but I still can't sleep." She paused, tearing up. "I'm short with my kids. I just worry so much I'm not being a good mom."

"I can understand that . . . like I can really relate," I said. "You know, parenting is the most difficult thing I've ever done. And as moms, we can be hard on ourselves. It's especially hard when you can't sleep."

"It's not just that," she said. "I cry for no reason. I don't think my medicine is working anymore."

Camila went on to describe her abdominal pain, which seemed to be contributing to her insomnia. She had cramping, bloating, and constipation, almost every day. Despite years of medical tests, diet changes, and medication trials, nothing really helped. Her history was consistent with irritable bowel syndrome, a common condition that, while not life-threatening, is often long-lasting and can impact quality of life.

"You're taking a pretty low dose of the antidepressant," I told her. "I think we should bump up the dose."

"Okay."

I paused. "I have another idea, too. . . . Have you ever tried meditation?" I was a little embarrassed to suggest it. It was outside the scope of my training. It certainly wasn't something I had learned about in medical school. But for someone with her symptoms and ongoing mood issues, it seemed like a good option.

"Well, I've heard of it," she said, "but I've never tried it."

"I've been learning a lot about it, and I think it might really help you," I said.

I couldn't do justice to the eight-week class in a short medical visit, but I hit a few highlights: the basic concept of mindfulness, using breath as an anchor, and body scan. We took some breaths together, slow, focused. I recommended a free app with various guided meditations.

A month later, she was better. Not totally better and not just because of meditation. We had upped her dose of antidepressants, and her food truck was enjoying some early success. But she had tried out the app and some of the breathing exercises. I was heartened by her progress and grateful for this new tool to offer those with chronic pain, depression, and anxiety.

﹏

At the end of our eight-week class, Geeta guided us through a full-day silent retreat. By that time, I was sold on the power of meditation. It had improved my stress, anxiety, and sleep. Most surprising, it had reduced my dizziness more than anything else.

We gathered early on a Sunday morning in our usual room and began a series of meditations, reviewing most of the types of meditation we had learned during the class. I sat still and focused on my breath, moved through gentle yoga positions, and walked barefoot and in slow motion around the courtyard, mindful of movement. Late in the morning, Geeta encouraged us to go a little farther from the room, and I wandered down to Lady Bird Lake, just a block away, and walked on the trail, looking, I'm sure, like a zombie.

We didn't speak or make eye contact, but I was glad Don was there, too. I even thought of that first raisin exercise when we ate lunch at Casa de Luz, in silence, noticing each bite of food—the various textures and flavors.

The experience of the silent retreat was like taking a final exam. I thought of Ella's upcoming ice-skating performance; after rehearsing for weeks, she would pull her skills together for the final show of the year. Except our grand finale meditation class lacked the stress and the need to prove mastery. We practiced all that we had learned, but there was no judge, no audience. There was only that one breath, one step, one moment. I had learned to sit still.

CHAPTER 33:

A Near Miss

March 2015

I couldn't sleep again. Although meditation had cured my long-standing insomnia, this was different: I was waking up in the middle of the night to jolts of heat, like jumping into a hot tub. When it happened, I would throw off the covers and stomp over to turn on the fan, angry that I had awakened. I would wipe my sweaty forehead and wait for the feeling to pass.

It had to be MS, right? Heat intolerance is common with the disease, though these sensations were waking me up and seemed to originate with me, not in response to a hot room. What else could it be?

I tried mindfulness techniques to get back to sleep, but my middle-of-the-night thoughts were insistent, intrusive. MS could cause practically anything. It wouldn't let me get too cozy and complacent. MS, the villain, would pop up whenever I started to think it was done with me, to imagine I had been set free. Now it was back, splashing me with boiling, blistering disappointment.

Until those new symptoms started, MS had stopped dominating my thoughts and dictating my life choices. My medication had protected me from relapses for almost five years. I had gotten used to stable MRIs with no new white spots. I had felt confident making big plans for my new clinic: expanded access to immunizations; universal screening for anxiety and depression with same-day, on-site counseling available; meditation classes for the staff. I was running longer loops with Jess, five miles, sometimes seven. I had planted my own plot in the community garden and looked forward to harvesting green beans, carrots, and tomatoes that summer. And I was planning adventurous trips with the kids—Colorado, maybe Hawaii?

Dr. Reynard and I would celebrate after each annual MRI.

"Another MRI without change!" he would say. "That's great news. The longer you go without progression, the less likely you are to have more MRI changes."

MS was like cancer in this regard; my prognosis improved with each relapse-free day. But, like cancer, it could always come back.

I decided to investigate. Were these sensory changes—feeling hot, minor night sweats—known signs of MS? The Internet said yes. I would need another MRI. But that was the last thing I wanted. All I could think of were the insurance hassles and time off from work, the loud banging of the machine and worrying about results. I didn't want to deal with that. And in my quest for an alternative explanation, I stumbled upon one so obvious that it made me laugh: *Could I be experiencing symptoms of menopause?*

I was only forty-one. I still had periods, though they were irregular. The average age for menopause is fifty-one. But I had just diagnosed a thirty-eight-year-old with premature ovarian failure, or early menopause. It was uncommon at my age, but possible. I, of all people, should know that.

I didn't call Dr. Reynard because I already had an appointment with my other doctor, an endocrinologist. I was scheduled to follow up on a thyroid nodule—a bump in my neck discovered one day while looking in the mirror and that, while benign, still required regular monitoring. A perpetual multitasker, I decided to ask my endocrinologist to add orders for my MS labs and a test for menopause to my routine thyroid bloodwork. If the labs showed I was in menopause, I could avoid an MRI and stop blaming MS.

My endocrinologist entered the room with a slight nod.

"How are you?" he asked. He did not shake hands or smile. He asked the question as if reading a script, in a monotone voice and with a coldness I had come to expect. He was the kind of doctor who expected to be called "Doctor" even by a fellow physician. He was formal, almost bored. But my thyroid issue was so minor, and I had been seeing him for so long, that I didn't want to bother switching doctors. I could tolerate this flat affect. Don and I would laugh about it later.

"I'm fine," I said. "How are you?"

He didn't answer. Instead, he scanned my thyroid ultrasound report.

"No growth of the nodule," he said.

"Okay, good to hear," I replied. "By the way, I'm having what I think could be hot flashes. I'm hoping you can order an FSH."

An FSH, or follicle-stimulating hormone, blood test can help to identify menopause in someone with characteristic symptoms. It could be done along with my routine MS and thyroid labs.

The endocrinologist didn't inquire about my symptoms. Had a forty-one-year-old patient mentioned having hot flashes to me, I would have bombarded her with questions: Do you have other symptoms? Are you still having periods? Are you using hormonal contraception? How old was your mom when she went through menopause?

I would have been curious. But although he agreed to the labs, he was uninterested.

He circled various test names and handed me the lab sheet. "Come back in one year."

And not a moment sooner, I thought.

I didn't hear back from the endocrinologist's office. After a week, I tried to call but got stuck in a phone tree that was almost as bad as the specialty pharmacy that delivered my MS medicine. I was finally able to leave a message, but the office didn't call me back. *Probably my labs were normal, and they didn't see a reason to call,* I thought. But I needed to be sure. Never trust anyone, never assume anything, I had learned from years of clinical practice.

I was swamped with work, coordinating schedules for the kids, trying to squeeze in time to meditate and exercise. But I needed to know if I was having an MS relapse or menopause. Maybe even my thyroid had become overactive and was causing my symptoms. Or something else could be wrong; night sweats, which sometimes accompanied my hot flashes, were seen with cancer, tuberculosis.

Nearly three weeks after my appointment, I called again.

"Thank you for calling. To make an appointment, please press 1."

I didn't wait for the other options because I figured my best bet to reach an actual person was to call the appointment desk. I pushed "1."

"We apologize, but all of our schedulers are occupied at the moment. Please leave a message."

"No!" I said aloud, slamming down the phone. "I already left a message. Goddamn it! Why can't you at least put me on hold?"

I hated to play the doctor card—it felt like cheating, cutting in line, an abuse of power—but I was fed up. I picked up the medical society directory and entered the number for the endocrinologist's secret backline into my phone. These confidential numbers were reserved for physician calls to request information or a consultation from the specialist. They weren't supposed to be used by patients, and in this case, I was the patient. *What does it matter if I break the rules?* I thought. *My doctor already seems to be mad at me—at the world—all the time.*

A nurse answered the phone. *A real person!*

"I'm so sorry to do this," I said. "I'm a doctor, but I'm actually calling as a patient on the backline because I couldn't get through on the main line. I need to get my own lab results."

The nurse wasn't overjoyed to talk to me, but she located my chart and results.

"Everything is normal," she said.

"Okay, great," I said, though I knew it wasn't great. If my labs were normal, I was probably having an MS relapse. I decided to double-check.

"So, the FSH . . . that was the lab I was most interested in . . . it's normal, too?"

She paused, presumably to look at the labs again. "An FSH wasn't done. I just see a CBC, CMP, and a TSH," she said, summarizing the other labs that had been ordered.

Really?

"Hmm . . . I'm surprised an FSH wasn't done. I saw it on the lab order sheet," I said.

She was silent for a minute. I waited, trying to control my exasperation.

"Oh! Here it is," she said at last. "It was on another screen in our electronic record. Yes, the FSH is normal."

"Good, I'm glad you found it. Can you give me the exact value of the FSH?" I was being *that* patient, second-guessing, irritating, impossible to satisfy. So be it.

Her answer justified my doubt, my paranoia.

"The FSH was fifty-three," she said, resigned to my entitled attitude.

Fifty-three! My mind did cartwheels and flip-flops. *Fifty-three is not normal! Fifty-three isn't even equivocal. What was she thinking?*

"Okay, well then, you've just diagnosed me with early menopause," I said. Now I was being a jerk, but I was livid. "I'm only forty-one. An FSH of fifty-three is consistent with menopause and is definitely not normal for my age."

"It shows that it's in the normal range," she said.

"The normal range for someone with menopause," I said. I asked her to mail me a copy of the results. I certainly wasn't going to rely on her interpretation. Then I made an appointment with my gynecologist to start treatment to stop the hot flashes.

I was struck with a mishmash of feelings. On the one hand, I was in menopause—or pretty darn close. The formal definition of menopause is the point in time when twelve months have passed since a woman's last period. Technically speaking, I was still in "perimenopause" —the menopausal transition—though likely close to the end of it. I was almost certainly infertile; I was old. I felt like I had crossed an invisible threshold to old age sooner than I should have. But—and this was a big but—I wasn't having MS progression. I also could count myself lucky since I wasn't having a lot of the other challenges many women, including some of my patients, face during perimenopause: heavy bleeding, mood changes, sleep disturbances, headaches, fatigue. I could deal with the hot flashes, especially since I now knew the cause. Because I certainly wasn't planning for more kids, early meno-pause seemed like the best-case scenario.

At the same time, I was enraged to think that my diagnosis was nearly missed. *If I hadn't called for the results (more than once) . . . if I had taken the nurse's word that everything was normal . . . if I hadn't asked specifically about the FSH result . . . if I hadn't been a doctor and known that an FSH of fifty-three was abnormal for a forty-one-year-old . . .*

In medicine, and probably in every other profession, the stagger-ing number of near-misses and real misses is overwhelming. A 2016 analysis by Johns Hopkins researchers concluded that medical error is the third leading cause of death in the United States, after heart disease and cancer. Medical errors include misdiagnosis, delayed diagnosis, medication errors, faulty medical devices, and especially communication problems.[1]

And what about people—like most of my patients at the new clinic—who didn't speak English? Those who couldn't read, had se-rious mental illness, or dementia? Those with disabilities? I thought of my patients who were blind, hearing-impaired, or couldn't walk. What about the people who didn't know how to advocate for them-selves, who felt uncomfortable questioning authority or didn't know they had a right to do so? There was no way that they were receiving the same quality of care that I, an educated white woman, with a med-ical degree to boot, was able to get.

Just a few weeks earlier, I had seen a new patient who reported a long-standing diagnosis of coronary artery disease. At her first visit, she shared her history of a heart attack three or four years earlier. She was in her late forties—young for a heart attack—but I prescribed as-pirin and cholesterol medicine to reduce her risk of another episode.

During the week after her visit, I also managed to dig up old medical records and pore through dozens of pages before I found what I was looking for: a heart catheterization report. And it was normal—no coronary artery blockages. She had not had a heart attack. I stopped the aspirin and cholesterol medicine. We rejoiced that, in her case, my double-checking led to good news.

I worried about all those abnormal x-rays, MRIs, lab tests, biopsy results, and lost hospital records that were lurking in the shadows. Nearly everyone I've talked to, in the years since, who has had any kind of major medical event, has a similar story to mine, but the known errors represent only a fraction of the total. I prided myself on follow-through for my patients, but my productivity and stress levels took a hit. Our system didn't reward diligence. Doctors were supposed to see more patients, not spend time reviewing records and chasing down test results. When I found a patient's old CT scan from the ER showing a lung mass or stumbled upon malignant melanoma on a well-woman exam, I didn't congratulate myself on the "good pickup." I worried about the inevitable misses.

Medical therapy reduced my hot flashes. But the experience reinforced the need for advocacy, both for my patients and myself. I would find a new endocrinology doctor for my thyroid. Though it meant more time at the clinic, I was motivated to spend even more time at the end of each day double- and triple-checking my patients' test results, reviewing old notes, and making sure they were notified of my findings and recommendations. And I was left with other lessons learned: be vigilant, cross your fingers, ask lots of questions, don't trust anyone. There were no good answers.

CHAPTER 34:

Cotton Balls

May 2015

One evening as I was getting ready for bed, I noticed an unusual sensation on the bottom of my foot. Stepping down on that foot felt like stepping on cotton balls. Maybe there was something wrong with my sock—the fabric was worn and uneven— or maybe something soft had found its way inside. I felt the bottom of my sock and then slipped it off. The sock was stretched out, but nothing was inside. When I set my foot down, the cotton ball remained.

Well, this is a new one, I thought. I went to bed and tried to forget about it.

The next day the cotton ball sensation was still there, and I thought maybe my other foot was a little numb as well. It wasn't unpleasant . . . *just another false alarm*, I thought. The hot flashes had been menopause. Weird tingling in my back the year before had turned out to be shingles—another diagnosis that, while unfortunate, still seemed far better than an MS flare. *I can live with the cotton balls,* I thought. *Plus, I've gone five years without disease progression. I never miss my medication. Surely, new MS activity is unlikely.* Granted, my job was even more stressful than I'd expected, but I was meditating twice a day and running more than ever. Clara didn't wake us up much anymore. And I wasn't convinced that stress was even connected with MS progression.

In the absence of anything dramatic, I watched my symptoms for several days without taking action. Remembering his reaction to Ella's visual complaints two years earlier, I also knew better than to tell Don. I knew my news would upset him at best, or it might lead to a full-scale panic attack if I misjudged my timing and his stress level.

The numbness was only bothersome because of what it might mean, not because it was painful or irritating itself. As it began to spread up my legs, I knew it must be a relapse. I wondered if I could wish it away. Was it really a big deal? Did I need to switch medicines for every relapse or just if I experienced really disabling symptoms?

As much as I hated to admit it, those weren't my only symptoms. My hands were starting to feel a little numb and tingly. Even more troubling were my bowel and bladder issues that were too embarrassing to discuss with anyone. I no longer thought they were just normal consequences of two pregnancies; MS had to be responsible. And maybe those hot flashes weren't just menopause after all.

I performed a mini neurologic exam on myself. My balance and strength seemed normal. I wasn't in pain. But I knew I should tell someone. Don deserved to know. He would make me call Dr. Reynard, which would trigger a necessary, but unwanted, chain reaction: an MRI, then bad news and disappointment—my five-year lucky streak would be broken—followed by a new medicine, a fight with my insurance company, and new side effects.

I agonized over what to do but tried to put it out of mind as I read *Harry Potter and the Sorcerer's Stone* to Clara that night. We were almost finished and were looking forward to the second book in the series.

"More!" Clara said, as I dog-eared the page and closed the book.

"We'll read tomorrow night, but now it's time to go to sleep."

I was glad Clara liked the book. She didn't have Ella's attention span, so getting her engaged in a story was more difficult. But she was sweet and thoughtful and still so young. As she snuggled with me, I was reminded that even if I didn't want to deal with MS for my own sake, I needed to for hers. And for Ella's and Don's.

I made up my mind. After tucking Clara into bed, I went back into my own bedroom and shared the news of my symptoms with Don, who reacted with reasonable but not excessive concern. The next day I called Dr. Reynard, who ordered an MRI of my entire spine. (I made sure of that, knowing the extent of my symptoms.) I went in for the test.

MS doesn't follow a playbook. With many other chronic diseases, the course is predictable, and the patient's actions can make a difference. With poor control of diabetes, for example, the kidneys and eyes are often affected, nerve damage can cause pain and numbness in the feet, and the risk of heart disease is increased. Diabetes can be a devastating disease, but affected patients have a measure of control. They can watch their diet, lose weight, and exercise to prevent the disease from worsening. The clinical course of MS, though, is more random. Healthy lifestyle still is important, especially to lower the chance of getting another chronic condition. But it may not slow disease progression. Medications are critical—the best way to lower risk of a relapse—and I took mine consistently. I had managed to fantasize that after five years with stable MRIs and strict adherence to "good health habits," I would continue to hold MS at bay, that I was in control. But back in the MRI tube, I felt certain this time that the news would not be good.

"Well, you called it," said the radiologist as we reviewed the films together in his dark office. I was right. The fact that the MRI validated my own suspicions—that I knew my body, and I could tell when the disease was back to wreak more havoc—was overshadowed by the two new white spots, bright and defiant, on the MRI pictures of my neck and lower back.

"A spinal lesion is worse than a brain lesion when it comes to predicting long-term disability," the radiologist explained. "One spinal lesion is equivalent to two brain lesions."

"It's crazy because I'm actually feeling so much better," I said. "My dizziness has improved."

"Well, that's good to hear, but I have no doubt your doctor will want to change your medication."

Okay, at least now I know. It's hard to accept, but it's out of my control. There's nothing I can do except follow up with my doctor and do what he says. I was resigned.

The confirmation of my relapse hit Don harder than me. While I was disappointed, I could cope. But Don became quiet and withdrawn, retreating to the couch after dinner, escaping into another crossword puzzle. I missed his silly jokes, his stories from work at the hospital. I wanted him to turn toward me, to grieve with me, and to provide reassurance. I also reprimanded myself for having any expectations, any dependency. *I am strong and self-sufficient. Why should I need anything from him?* But I did. I needed him. I felt deserted, lonely. I wanted him to check in with me, be interested in my reaction, show concern mixed with optimism.

He couldn't do it.

Looking back now, I can see that he had a right to his shock, even if I would have appreciated a more stoic response. I had lived with my new symptoms for a while, slowly getting used to the idea of a relapse, like gradually easing into a bath full of ice cubes or the popular and famously cold Barton Springs Pool near downtown Austin. I didn't tell Don about my symptoms for days, maybe weeks, knowing he might panic. I didn't give him long to prepare for the finality of the MRI. Instead, I pushed him headfirst into the icy water.

In the two weeks between the MRI and my appointment with Dr. Reynard, we distracted ourselves with work and the kids. Don was anxious, but my new job was so busy and overwhelming that I didn't have time to think about MS, the MRI, Don's reaction, or anything else. When we finally discussed my upcoming visit with Dr. Reynard, I assumed Don would want to come. He didn't.

"I can't do anything to help. My being there won't change anything," he argued.

"You're not curious, like to hear what he wants to do?" I asked.

"Well, sure, but you can fill me in later," he said.

Despite my efforts to reframe his reaction, to tell myself that his panic was actually a sign of his concern and affection for me, I was angry.

"So, this sucks and is scary, and you don't want to deal with it?" I asked the night before the appointment. "Well, it sounds like the perfect solution for you is to bail, and I'll go deal with it all alone. That's the foundation of a happy and supportive marriage after all."

"I'll go if you want me to," he said.

"If I *want* you to?"

"I just don't see the point since there's nothing I can do."

"Uh, support me? Hold my hand? Comfort me as I'm hearing bad news and making a hard decision about my next steps?"

"It sounds like you want me to come," he said.

My husband. Master of subtlety. "Not if it's going to be such a burden for you and wreck your day," I said. "But yes, I think you should come. I think I shouldn't have to ask you. You should be there as my partner and my friend."

By morning, my anger had subsided along with Don's resistance. Of course, he would come. I shouldn't have needed to persuade him. Sometimes he was my rock, and sometimes he was my rockslide. But as we drove to Dr. Reynard's office, I realized the avalanche had stopped, and we walked into the office as a team.

The exam room felt cold. I sat next to Don in a chair against the wall, waiting for Dr. Reynard. We didn't talk. I buttoned the top buttons on my sweater. I crossed and uncrossed my legs. We both scrolled through messages and articles on our phones. I couldn't concentrate on my e-mails. I would have to read them all again later.

The appointment did not have the celebratory tone of visits from the past few years. There was no "Congratulations! You're still relapse-free." Dr. Reynard had said that the longer I went without disease progression, the less likely I was to have further relapses. Of course, the corollary to his statement was that my new symptoms and MRI changes now made future deterioration much more likely.

"Hello again," Dr. Reynard said as he entered the room and shook our hands. "I know you're aware of your results, but let's go over the MRI together and discuss the options."

Dr. Reynard pulled up the MRI on his computer screen, and we studied the pictures together. *How doomed am I?* Dr. Reynard flipped through the screens, orienting us to the anatomy I was supposed to know but always forgot, and pointing out the changes he saw. Two new spinal lesions were the biggest concern.

"The location of the lesions corresponds with your symptoms," he said. "And I still don't see any black holes. At least that's one bit of good news."

"Do I definitely have to switch meds?" I asked. "I know about the new white spots on the MRI, but if there are no black holes and if my symptoms are tolerable, is it really essential?"

"No question really," he said. "Often people will fail the injectable medicines after a period of time. It would be safer to change, and there are a couple of options."

I jotted down notes as Dr. Reynard reviewed my choices: I could start IV infusion treatment with a medicine I had rejected in the past because of serious health risks or try a new oral medication that was not quite as effective but not quite as risky. To help make the decision, I needed a blood test that was now available to assess my risk of PML, that terminal brain disease that was known to occur, in rare instances, with the first medicine. If the test was positive, my risk increased from less than one in a thousand to nearly one in a hundred.

I went that afternoon to the lab, and the following week I heard the news: The test was positive. I wouldn't be a good candidate for the infusion therapy. The oral option, Dr. Reynard said, would be my best bet.

⌐⁓

Almost as much as I resented the new white spots, I dreaded the next steps in adjusting my treatment plan: the additional doctor visits (an eye exam and dermatology visit were required), clashes with my insurance company, more blood tests, an electrocardiogram, long phone trees to connect with new specialty pharmacies. Dr. Reynard couldn't just write me a prescription to start the new medicine the next day. It would take months to make the change. If I elected to start the new medicine, a doctor would have to come to my house for an entire day to administer my first dose and monitor me to make sure my heart rate didn't drop too low.

I was able to read about MS now. I was like a ten-year-old, seeing the horror movie *Poltergeist* for a second time and daring myself not to cover my eyes again, to be brave and watch the whole thing. And now the news on MS was encouraging. New studies would pop up sometimes in my family medicine journals and newsletters, providing more clues to the causes of MS, describing the latest medications and other treatments. I even sought out continuing medical education activities on multiple sclerosis and attended a conference where Dr. Reynard was giving a lecture.

Even though I knew I could face the studies and review articles about MS medications, I surprised myself with delay tactics that kept me from researching my new treatment. While I told Dr. Reynard to proceed with the prior authorization process with my insurance company, and I scheduled the required ophthalmology and dermatology appointments, I felt I needed to learn about the medicine he was recommending to make sure it was the right choice.

I am the opposite of a procrastinator. I usually do unpleasant tasks first because I am gratified by the delay of gratification. I used to save my Halloween candy as a kid until it went bad, more satisfied with saving than consuming it. But this time, I just kept taking my old medication, and I put off doing the research as long as I could.

My job had again become all-consuming. I was now working more hours than ever and coping with a longer commute. I loved my patients at the new clinic, but their needs were almost too much to bear: a woman in her mid-forties slowly declining from early-onset dementia, a young man with inexplicable kidney failure, an older woman with terribly uncontrolled diabetes who rejected my pleas to start insulin. I was too caught up in their stories—and new administrative and staffing challenges I faced as medical director—to prioritize my own health concerns.

Ultimately I made myself investigate the options—at least a little. It felt hypocritical to dole out advice all day to my patients when I wasn't willing to follow my own doctor's advice. I turned to resources I used at the clinic, and even managed to consult another MS specialist through an online tool I could access through my work. I learned about a different medicine—one that was perhaps equally effective and less risky than the one that Dr. Reynard had recommended.

At our next visit, still waiting for the pieces to fall into place for me to get my new medicine, I admitted to Dr. Reynard that I had been doing more research, including the virtual second opinion.

"So why not this other medicine? Is it safer than what you're proposing?" I asked.

"The hurdles are not insignificant for the medicine I'm recommending," Dr. Reynard said. "I think that may be the reason some doctors don't want to start it. But newer studies are showing it is a more effective option. And if you can get over the obstacles of initiation, it's actually better tolerated."

"But it's a new medicine. I'm worried about the cancer risk and possible heart problems," I said.

"It's been on the market for nearly six years. It's been well studied."

"Yes, but there are so many medicines that have been out there for years that I've prescribed to my patients. Then years or even decades later, we discover new risks. Newer medicines are always the riskiest," I said.

I thought of a common diabetes medicine that was later linked to heart attacks, hormonal treatment for menopause found to increase the risk of breast cancer, certain medicines for acid reflux associated with pneumonia. Again, I suggested sticking with my current treatment. "I mean, I don't like giving myself the injections, but I'm used to it by now. Is it really not working just because it didn't stop this one relapse?"

"It's not a risk I'd want to take," he said. "We have a better medicine now. You're a good candidate for it. Read about it. I think you will feel better doing some additional research."

I suspected my doctor was impatient with me—hell, I was impatient with me. The odds of further MS progression increased each day I delayed my decision. Finally, one evening, I ran out of excuses. Forcing myself to sit down in front of my laptop, I did what I should have done in the first place. I logged into UpToDate, a subscription service that had effectively replaced *Harrison's Principles of Internal Medicine* as the premiere go-to reference for clinical information. And Dr. Reynard was right—I felt better. The safety profile was reasonable: side effects were few, long-term risks seemed small. The alternatives looked worse. It was a sound choice, and I would do it.

During the next several weeks, I fretted with the insurance company, wondering why the process for approval had to be so cumbersome. But then again, the new medicine, like many MS drugs, was priced at over sixty thousand dollars a year. They couldn't possibly want to make it easy for me. I reminded myself that I was fortunate to have insurance in the first place. I couldn't imagine trying to start the same medication for one of my uninsured patients.

Even with my advantages, the challenges continued. After waiting weeks for an appointment, my records from the ophthalmologist were lost in the process of being sent to Dr. Reynard's office. Only when Dr. Reynard's medical assistant, as a very special favor to me, drove to the ophthalmologist's office in person were the records finally placed in the right hands. Meanwhile, I continued the same medicine, knowing each delay was potentially jeopardizing my health.

A week before the Big Day, when I would receive the first dose of my new medicine in my home under the watchful eye of a visiting physician and his medical assistant, I still wasn't sure if I could put all the pieces together to make it happen.

"Thank you for your call. We are experiencing an unusually heavy call volume at this time. We appreciate your patience."

I heard that same greeting, over and over again, as I tried, after morning clinic and before my afternoon meetings began, to contact the mail-order specialty pharmacy, the insurance company, the drug manufacturer's assistance program that covered my (large) co-pay, and Dr. Reynard's office, to ensure that my medicine was approved and would arrive by the next morning. Each person I talked to told me to call another place; no one seemed to have talked to anyone else. Flustered and bewildered, I felt like a ball in a game of doubles ping-pong.

"Look," I said to the insurance agent during our second call. "You told me to call the mail-order pharmacy, they told me to call the co-pay assistance program, and they told me to call you. I am running around in circles, and I just want to be sure this medicine gets delivered on time."

"I understand, but the pharmacy is in charge of ensuring timely delivery."

"Yes, I get that. But they say that there is some issue with the co-pay assistance, and the co-pay assistance says they need some kind of approval or confirmation from you." I was totally exasperated.

"We have provided that," said the insurance agent.

"Okay, good. So can you please call the pharmacy and tell them that? I'd like to stay on the phone and make sure we are all on the same page," I said.

To my relief, the agent agreed. She initiated a three-way call with the pharmacy, sorted out the issues with the co-pay assistance and delivery, and assured me the medicine would arrive. I was equal parts relieved and furious, appalled that everything needed to be so damn complicated.

When the medicine was delivered the next morning, I opened the cardboard box to find an unassuming plastic container. *All that trouble for these little pills*, I thought.

After dropping the kids at summer camp, I greeted the internal medicine doctor and his medical assistant, welcoming them to my living room to set up shop. This small team was charged with spending six hours observing and monitoring me after I popped that first pill. I was grateful they could come to my home, where I could work between my blood pressure checks and heart exams.

The doctor ran an electrocardiogram to assess my heart rhythm and function, and I swallowed the first $170 capsule.

"How often have you had to resuscitate someone?" I asked the doctor after exchanging the usual pleasantries and swapping backstories about where we went to medical school and completed our residency training. "Have you actually had anyone go into heart block or have an arrhythmia?"

"Not so far," he answered.

"Well, I don't want to be the first," I said.

A couple of hours after I took the medicine, my heart rate dropped by twenty beats per minute but was still in the normal range. I felt a vague dizziness, but otherwise I was fine. I worked. Don sent check-in texts every hour or two, and I answered that everything was okay. The medical assistant monitored and recorded my pulse and blood pressure every hour. A friend, Naomi Hanser—the doctor I'd hired at my previous clinic a couple years earlier—brought vegan wraps from Conscious Cravings for lunch.

"Well, I think you're good to go," said the doctor, at the end of our six-hour observation period. "Good luck with the new med."

"Thanks," I said.

All that rigmarole, and now we were done. Time to rekindle hope and move on.

CHAPTER 35:

The Finish Line

September 2015

I didn't tell anyone I was training for a marathon. I couldn't even commit to it myself. A marathon had always seemed impossible. It wasn't something *I* could do, plus I had other hobbies and goals. Though I envied my friends who trained, I told myself I was too slow, too busy, too likely to get injured. My time was better spent on work, organizing the house, carting the kids to school and activities.

But in the months after starting my new medicine, a marathon seemed to reveal itself on my bucket list. I think it had been there all along, written in invisible ink, and now I was starting to see it, not sure if I wanted to erase it or move it to the top of the list. Because I couldn't make up my mind, I continued to run as I always had. I just ran a little farther every weekend—to keep my options open—until the marathon became almost inevitable.

Always beautiful, the lake revealed subtle changes every week. The color usually mirrored the sky—shades of blue or gray—but could be a muddy brown after a storm when the rain left big puddles on the trail. By early fall, the leaves were still green but tired. A gang of four loud, rambunctious geese often clustered together near the cypress trees, threatening any runner or excited dog that got too close. The little ducks from Canada—the black and white coots—would soon start gathering with the turtles near the gazebo, hoping to be fed.

At least once a week, Jess met me and my dog, Clover, at the lake. Our running sessions were part exercise, part therapy: parent coaching, marriage counseling, health advice. Each time we met, we took turns recounting the latest episode of our lives. Sometimes it was a sitcom, other times a drama; usually it was a little of both. We could have met at a coffee shop, but as Jess said, we were multitasking by exercising while we talked. I loved these runs, and we were always surprised by how fast the time passed.

"How was the week?" she asked one Sunday morning in late September as we started off on the footbridge, crossing over the lake. The water was like glass, reflecting the early-morning light, with a single rower breaking the surface in a narrow line.

"Too busy. I'm working ridiculous hours at the clinic, and I can't fit everything in. But I guess that's what I say every week," I said.

We darted around an older couple and settled behind a group of college students who ran in a tight cluster, much faster than we would ever be.

"Yes, but I think it's inevitable right now," she said. "You're working full-time. Our kids may be in upper elementary school, but they still need a lot."

"Right? I mean, each year gets a little easier, but it's never actually *easy*," I said. "I have a friend from medical school with three kids who just got her MBA . . . in her spare time. She works full-time, too. Imagine!"

"I don't know how some people do it," she said. "But you're doing a lot. Give yourself some credit."

As usual, her words were reassuring. Jess—a treasured part of my support circle—was always there to listen to my struggles and share her own.

"Thanks. I know I complain about being overwhelmed all the time, but it's really a good problem to have. It's a gift to never be bored, to have a life that's too full," I said.

We ran under a canopy of leaves, and I ducked to avoid a stray vine.

"How far are you running today?" she asked. "I think I'm up for about five miles."

"I'm aiming for ten," I said. "We can run the five-mile loop together, and then I can run it a second time by myself . . . well, with Clover."

As my goal took shape, I treasured it as a secret, a fantasy I could consider and revise without judgment. If I didn't tell anyone, I could change my mind without having to explain anything. I didn't want to reveal it unless I felt certain I could do it.

I imagined Don would complain, criticize, try to talk me out of it. *Are you insane?* I thought he would say. It was too far, too stressful, too time-consuming. I already complained about my too-long to-do list. But I kept adding one mile to my long run every week or two: six miles, then seven, eight, now ten.

When I got to eleven or twelve, Jess made me fess up. I had hinted at the possibility of a marathon some weeks before, but I had remained noncommittal.

"It seems like you're really going to do this," she said one Saturday, just as we crossed the footbridge and turned to run along the south side of the lake. "What's your plan at this point?"

"I'm still not sure," I answered. Clover darted ahead as I marveled at the cool autumn weather that had finally replaced the oppressive summer heat.

"Have you thought of joining a training program?"

"Not really. I don't want to commit to that. I'm just adding a mile a week to the long runs," I said. She was the only one who knew.

"Why do you want to do it?" she asked.

"I'm still not sure I do, but I guess because I want to prove to myself that I can. I'm over forty now. I have MS. I don't know how long I'll be in good enough shape to even consider it."

"Well, twenty-six miles is more than I'd ever want to run, but I guess that makes sense," she said, adjusting her baseball cap.

Jess convinced me to meet with a trainer—she arranged it, joined me for the consultation, and even split the cost. The marathon was just two and a half months away. I hadn't registered. I hadn't talked to my family. But I came away from the session with a personalized training schedule, running advice, a video of cool-down stretches, and a conviction that, just maybe, I could do it.

Around that time, I finally confessed my marathon plan to Don. The secret was becoming too big to keep. And the time commitment was only going to increase. He needed to know.

Driving to my parents' house for a family dinner one evening—both kids now able to sit calmly, without car seats, in the back seat—I told him. "I ran fourteen miles today. It's the farthest I've ever run—seems like maybe I'm really going to run the marathon."

"Okay."

"Really? You're okay with that? I'm still not 100 percent, but I met with a trainer, and I'm following the schedule. It actually seems doable."

"Sure. You're the one running it. You're not asking me to do it."

"I thought you'd be mad," I said.

"Why would I be mad? You can do what you want."

He didn't exactly encourage me, but his reaction was a relief. He didn't think I was crazy or selfish, even though I thought I was a little bit of both. Running a marathon wasn't helping anyone else. Maybe it would be good for my morale—proof that MS hadn't won. But I wasn't even running to raise money for a charity or for any purpose other than to say I could do it. I was taking away time from Don and the kids to train, to be alone or with my friend and my dog, running around the lake. At least the sense of accomplishment, the improvements to my mood and even my dizziness, meant that I was more present, more patient, and more positive with my family, with everyone.

Marathon training felt like the one aspect of my life that I could control. It was a break from the uncertainty I faced with my illness and, increasingly, with my career. MS relapses, job struggles, and middle-school decisions for Ella created an anxiety that brought back my insomnia in the middle of the night. But the marathon was a challenge that used to seem impossible and now was within my grasp, my pride growing each time I beat my last record for my farthest run.

The day of the marathon I awoke early, before my alarm, dressing in the dark and forcing myself to eat a banana with peanut butter, though I had no appetite. My pink-orange running shirt would make me easy to spot in the crowd when Don and the kids came to root for me. I clipped back my hair, applied sunscreen, and tied my Brooks tennis shoes with double knots.

Don drove me to the starting line through deserted streets that grew more crowded as we approached the Texas Capitol—the starting point for the race.

"You've got your iPod?" he asked.

"Yep. I can't wait to hear the mix you made."

"Okay. I'll see you at the nineteen-mile marker, and then at mile twenty-five," he reviewed.

"Can't wait, though I imagine I'm going to be ready to fall over and die by then."

"Good luck!"

He kissed me goodbye, and I went to join the masses of fellow marathon runners, lining the grounds of the Capitol, stretching, and chatting in the dim morning light.

I ran the first mile with tears streaming down my face. I was there, running a marathon, despite MS, and maybe because of it, too. Don's music accompanied me, reminding me of our first conversation in that Boston fraternity house nearly twenty-five years before. Nirvana, U2, REM, and Rush's "Dreamline," "Time Stand Still," and "Marathon"—each song was a message from him, encouraging me to go on as I ran down Congress Avenue, across the bridge, and over the lake: my lake.

People lined the streets, holding signs, cheering us on. It was Valentine's Day, and some people held up big red hearts cut out of poster board. I saw a pair of fellow runners wearing hot pink tutus. Frequently I pulled out my earbuds so I could hear a band or a solo musician that played on the side of road. Austin is, after all, known as the Live Music Capital of the World. On marathon day, it would live up to that name.

I loved the encouragement from the onlookers and laughed at their signs that said, "Great Job, Random Stranger," and "Run like there's a hot guy ahead of you and a creepy one behind you." "Free High Fives" read one sign, as I scooted to the side and high-fived a line of kids. I chuckled at "You're Running Better Than the Government," adding "and our health care system" under my breath. "Pain Now, Pride Forever" was another one that made me smile through tears.

I was running faster than usual, but I didn't want to slow down as I raced through South Austin and then back toward downtown, across the lake again and along the road that parallels my usual running path. I was not a great runner—I had never won a race, never run cross-country, never run a six-minute mile or even an eight-minute mile. I used to struggle to run the three-mile loop at the lake. Back then, six miles was a long run. I had convinced myself I would never, could never, run a marathon. But I had taken on the challenge, and now I was running, well trained, injury-free, and sure I could make it.

The challenge, I realized, didn't have to be a marathon. It could be anything. I just needed a tangible goal. Moving forward, if I lost my ability to run, perhaps I would swim or race in a wheelchair. If someday I couldn't work as a doctor, perhaps I would write or paint. Even if I was as incapacitated as Mr. Sloane, I would find a new "marathon" to match my abilities, to push my limits. I made a promise to myself to always set and work toward the next suitable goal that would provide a sense of purpose and accomplishment, even if I had restrictions.

Jess joined me for the last ten miles—the hardest ten miles I had ever run.

"How are you feeling?" she asked.

"My legs are numb, and I'm completely worn-out," I said.

"You were running fast," Jess noted. "I could track you on the marathon app, and I kept trying to send you psychic messages to slow down."

I mustered a soft laugh as we continued to trudge along a street near my old high school, north of downtown. We were heading back toward the university and then the Capitol. I managed to give a thumbs-up to a musician playing his harmonica on a corner as we passed.

"I felt so great for the first half, but I think I hit a wall around mile fourteen or fifteen. I'll be okay, though."

After an enthusiastic start, I was beat. I had slowed down by then, and I stopped to walk for a precious minute, to catch my breath, at every mile marker—a recommendation from the trainer. Jess had saved up stories to entertain and distract me, and she reminded me to get water, to eat another energy cube. Though she didn't have to remind me when it was time for our one-minute walk, she slowed her pace to be in sync with my own and then sped up again with me when the minute ended.

At mile nineteen, when we saw Don with ten-year-old Ella and eight-year-old Clara, I stopped for a five-second hug. I smiled at Clara's homemade sign: "Go, Mom!"

"You look great!" Don said. "Keep it up!"

At mile twenty-five, Don and the kids found us again, and Ella joined us.

"You're doing great, Mom," she said. I loved her encouragement as we jogged through downtown Austin, the crowds growing in size and volume as we neared the end. My pace was barely faster than a walk—too slow for Ella. The day had warmed up, and it was humid, sapping any remaining energy. But my daughter matched my step and ran beside me as we neared the Capitol.

One foot in front of the other. I'm in pain, but this is the way it is right now.

I couldn't talk anymore, but I managed a groan at the sight of the hill on San Jacinto, soon after passing the parking garage. I knew it was small, but it looked enormous. We started up.

"We're almost there," Jess said. "You're going to make it."

Thank God.

The slight downhill after turning onto 11th Street was more than welcome. I couldn't see the large green banner marking the finish line yet, but I knew we'd spot it just after the final left turn, back onto Congress Avenue.

People were crowded on both sides of the street, shouting, whistling, clapping, excited. Someone was pounding on a drum. "You're almost there!" "You can do it!"

"There it is," Ella said as we neared the corner of 11th and Congress. "Austin Marathon & Half Marathon" was written across the top of the banner, with green posts on either side, holding it up. I could make out my parents and Cathy just after the finish line. When they saw us, Cathy jumped up and down, and they all cheered—"Go, Lisa!" "You got this!"—prompting me to quicken my pace. With Ella and Jess beside me, I sprinted the final fifty yards before collapsing into the arms of my family in a series of sweaty hugs. Someone put a marathon "finisher" medal around my neck, and Cathy handed me a smoothie from Juiceland. I knew Don and Clara were parking the car and would join us soon. My favorite people. All there to support me—through anything. I felt triumphant. I knew I would still have to contend with

MS, but in that moment, I had beaten it. I could summon that courage and grit again. Persistence, fortitude. I had it in me, and I knew it.

Epilogue

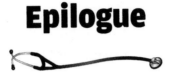

MS has added a bizarre twist to my quest to find fulfillment and to serve others. At times, it has helped me understand my purpose with greater clarity even while sometimes thwarting my plans. My focus has changed over time, adjusting itself to my whims, health limitations, and my family's interests and needs. I am thankful for each formation it has taken: the clinic, my patients, the marathon, my kids, this book.

Don is nostalgic for the days when Ella and Clara hugged him without prompting and snuggled with him before bed. I am not. Well, mostly not. Perhaps because my MS—with chronic dizziness and insomnia—plagued me for several years nearly every day, I don't remember with fondness those years of parenting young children.

I am grateful now that Ella prepares her own breakfast and lunch, drives herself to school, does her homework without prompting. But I am especially grateful for her generous spirit, friendly personality, remarkable sense of humor, her love of music and travel, her curiosity about the world. Despite my enormous inadequacies as her mother, she is okay—more than okay.

Clara doesn't wake us up in the middle of the night anymore. She is thoughtful, fiercely independent, and well loved by anyone who knows her. She is an excellent swimmer and gifted artist and photographer. She loves to play classic rock on Don's old electric guitar. Don and I no longer feel like we are in Dr. Seuss's Waiting Place. We are able to celebrate the place where we are now.

I don't exactly accept my MS. I still resent it. But I'm encouraged by the rapid advances in MS research and care that have led to new treatment approaches and a better understanding of the disease. And I have found ways to cope. Diet changes didn't help but stopping caffeine did. Continued meditation and mindfulness have helped reduce my anxiety about the future. Eternally frustrated with the health care system, as both a doctor and a patient, I left clinical practice to work for several years on programs to improve and transform the way health care is delivered at a population level. Although I missed my patients, I found a better balance for myself and my family. I have far more normal than dizzy days now. When, in late 2016, I had another flare, I switched medicines again and finished a draft of this book. I reminded myself, *this is the way it is right now.* I've had no detectable disease progression since. And another career shift, to include some direct patient care, is on the horizon.

MS is an excuse to sleep eight hours, even when I have too much to do. I prioritize self-care and remain vigilant about daily exercise. And MS has helped me confront mortality and form a tense alliance with uncertainty. I have also connected with the MS community by participating in the National MS Society's Texas MS150 every spring—a two-day bike ride, over 150 miles, which brings people together to raise awareness and funds to fight MS.

On the other hand, my concern about the U.S. health care

system—exacerbated by the COVID pandemic—continues unabated. Millions remain uninsured, and the situation in Texas is worse than any other state. I read their stories in news reports, and I see the impact during my regular volunteer sessions at a clinic for people experiencing homelessness. A report published in January 2023 by the Commonwealth Fund, comparing the United States to other high-income countries, shows that people in the United States face the worst health outcomes—with the lowest life expectancy and the highest death rates for treatable or preventable conditions. Despite spending the most per capita and as a percent of gross domestic product, the United States is the only nation that does not guarantee universal health coverage.[1]

Fortunately, I've discovered ways through my work and out-of-work activities to think creatively about system improvements, designing programs to support vulnerable populations and, most recently, joining a multidisciplinary team to improve care for people with multiple sclerosis in Central Texas. I also tackle big-picture issues, like climate change and pollution, in my work with Texas Physicians for Social Responsibility. My life is still as packed as an overstuffed suitcase, and I'm trying to make peace with that.

Life is like a coral reef, crafted from millions of moments instead of calcium deposits. It's haphazard and unpredictable, but that fragility contributes to its beauty. I am more aware of each moment now. MS has helped me appreciate them all.

Endnotes

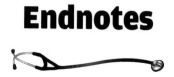

Chapter 2: Caring for Our Own

1. Jennifer Tolbert, Patrick Drake, and Anthony Damico, "Key Facts About the Uninsured Population," Kaiser Family Foundation, December 19, 2022, https://www.kff.org/uninsured/issue-brief/key-facts-about-the-uninsured-population/.

2. Families USA, "Dying for Coverage: The Deadly Consequences of Being Uninsured," June 2012, https://familiesusa.org/wp-content/up-loads/2019/09/Dying-for-Coverage.pdf.

3. Rachel Nuwer, "Universal Health Care Could Have Saved More Than 330,000 U.S. Lives During COVID," *Scientific American*, June 13, 2022, https://www.scientificamerican.com/article/universal-health-care-could-have-saved-more-than-330-000-u-s-lives-during-covid/.

4. Melanie Evans, Anna Wilde Mathews, and Tom McGinty, "Hospitals Often Charge Uninsured People the Highest Prices, New Data Show," *Wall Street Journal*, July 6, 2021, https://www.wsj.com/articles/hospitals-often-charge-uninsured-people-the-highest-prices-new-data-show-11625584448?mod=hp_lead_pos5.

Chapter 4: Worthy Pursuits

1. Centers for Disease Control and Prevention, "Diabetes Fast Facts," September 30, 2022, https://www.cdc.gov/diabetes/basics/quick-facts.html.

Chapter 5: Striving for Perfection

1. Robert M. A. Hirschfeld, Janet B. W. Williams, Robert L. Spitzer, Joseph R. Calabrese, Laurie Flynn, Paul E. Keck, Jr., Lydia Lewis, Susan L. McElroy, Robert M. Post, Daniel J. Rapport, James M. Russell, Gary S. Sachs, and John Zajecka, "Development and Validation of a Screening Instrument for Bipolar Spectrum Disorder: The Mood Disorder Questionnaire," *American Journal of Psychiatry* 157, no. 11(November 2000): 1873–1875, https://ajp.psychiatryonline.org/doi/epdf/10.1176/appi.ajp.157.11.1873.

2. Depression and Bipolar Support Alliance, "Bipolar Disorder Statistics," accessed February 19, 2023, https://www.dbsalliance.org/education/bipolar-disorder/bipolar-disorder-statistics/.

3. Peter Dome, Zoltan Rihmer, and Xenia Gonda, "Suicide Risk in Bipolar Disorder: A Brief Review," *Medicina* 55, no. 8 (July 24, 2019), https://www.ncbi.nlm.nih.gov/pmc/articles/PMC6723289/.

4. Mental Health America, "Access to Care Data 2022," accessed February 19, 2023, https://mhanational.org/issues/2022/mental-health-america-access-care-data.

Chapter 6: Something Bad

1. Toshi A. Furukawa, Andrea Cipriani, Lauren Z. Atkinson, Stefan Leucht, Yusuke Ogawa, Nozomi Takeshima, Yu Hayasaka, Anna Chaimani, and Georgia Salanti, "Placebo Response Rates in Antidepressant Trials: A Systematic Review of Published and Unpublished Double-Blind Randomised Controlled Studies," *Lancet Psychiatry* 3, no. 11 (November 2016): 1059–1066.

2. Mallika Marshall, "A Placebo Can Work Even When You Know It's a Placebo," Harvard Health Blog, July 7, 2016, https://www.health.harvard.edu/blog/placebo-can-work-even-know-placebo-201607079926.

3. Darcy Lockman, "Don't Be Grateful That Dad Does His Share," *The Atlantic,* May 7, 2019, https://www.theatlantic.com/ideas/archive/2019/05/mothers-shouldnt-be-grateful-their-husbands-help/588787/.

4. Paige Nong, Minakshi Raj, Melissa Creary, Sharon L. R. Kardia, and Jodyn E. Platt, "Patient-Reported Experiences of Discrimination in the US Health Care System," *JAMA Network Open* 3, no. 12 (December 15, 2020): e2029650, https://jamanetwork.com/journals/jamanetworkopen/

fullarticle/2774166.

Chapter 7: White Spots

1. Mitchell T. Wallin, William J. Culpepper, Jonathan D. Campbell, Lorene M. Nelson, Annette Langer-Gould, Ruth Ann Marrie, Gary R. Cutter, Wendy E. Kaye, Laurie Wagner, Helen Tremlett, Stephen L. Buka, Piyameth Dilokthornsakul, Barbara Topol, Lie H. Chen, and Nicholas G. LaRocca, "The Prevalence of MS in the United States: A Population-Based Estimate Using Health Claims Data," *Neurology* 92, no. 10 (March 5, 2019): e1029-e1040, https://n.neurology.org/content/92/10/e1029.

Chapter 12: Out of Control

1. American Psychological Association, "Stress a Major Health Problem in the U.S., Warns APA," 2007, https://www.apa.org/news/press/releases/2007/10/stress.

2. American Psychological Association, "APA: U.S. Adults Report Highest Stress Level Since Early Days of the COVID-19 Pandemic," February 2, 2021, https://www.apa.org/news/press/releases/2021/02/adults-stress-pandemic.

Chapter 13: Diseases That Really Suck

1. Centers for Disease Control and Prevention, "Working Together to Reduce Black Maternal Mortality," April 6, 2022, https://www.cdc.gov/healthequity/features/maternal-mortality/index.html.

2. Latoya Hill and Samantha Artiga, "COVID-19 Cases and Deaths by Race/Ethnicity: Current Data and Changes over Time," Kaiser Family Foundation, August 22, 2022, https://www.kff.org/coronavirus-covid-19/issue-brief/covid-19-cases-and-deaths-by-race-ethnicity-current-data-and-changes-over-time/#:~:text=It%20finds%3A,age%20by%20race%20and%20ethnicity.

3. Centers for Disease Control and Prevention, Alzheimer's Disease and Healthy Aging, "Loneliness and Social Isolation Linked to Serious Health Conditions," last updated April 29, 2021, https://www.cdc.gov/aging/publications/features/lonely-older-adults.html.

Chapter 14: Whac-A-Mole

1. Office of the National Coordinator for Health Information Technology, "Office-Based Physician Electronic Health Record Adoption," Health IT Quick-Stat 50, accessed February 19, 2023, https://www.healthit.gov/data/quickstats/office-based-physician-electronic-health-record-adoption.

Chapter 15: The Waiting Place

1. Dr. Seuss, *Oh, the Places You'll Go!* New York: Random House, 1990, n.p.

Chapter 16: Another Catch-22

1. Centers for Disease Control and Prevention, "Deaths from Excessive Alcohol Use in the United States," July 6, 2022, https://www.cdc.gov/alcohol/features/excessive-alcohol-deaths.html#:~:text=More%20than%20140%2C000%20people%20die,in%20the%20U.S.%20each%20year.

Chapter 17: Back So Soon?

1. Yuzhu Li, Barbara J. Sahakian, Jujiao Kang, et al., "The Brain Structure and Genetic Mechanisms Underlying the Nonlinear Association Between Sleep Duration, Cognition, and Mental Health," *Nature Aging* 2 (April 28, 2022): 425–437, https://doi.org/10.1038/s43587-022-00210-2.

Chapter 18: An Ill-Equipped Life Raft

1. American Psychiatric Association, "Mental Health Disparities: Diverse Populations," 2017, https://www.psychiatry.org/File%20Library/Psychiatrists/Cultural-Competency/Mental-Health-Disparities/Mental-Health-Facts-for-Diverse-Populations.pdf.

Chapter 23: From Clueless to Competent

1. Melinda Magyari and Per Soelberg Sorensen, "Comorbidity in Multiple Sclerosis," *Frontiers in Neurology* 11 (August 21, 2020): 851, doi: 10.3389/fneur.2020.00851.

Chapter 25: The Renovation

1. Justin Porter, Cynthia Boyd, M. Reza Skandari, et al., "Revisiting the Time Needed to Provide Adult Primary Care," *Journal of General Internal Medicine* 38 (2023): 147–155, https://doi.org/10.1007/s11606-022-07707-x.

Chapter 27: You Win Some, You Lose Some

1. Dan Wagener, ed., "Alcoholics Anonymous: The 12 Steps of AA & Success Rates," American Addiction Centers, February 2, 2023, https:// americanaddictioncenters.org/rehab-guide/12-step/whats-the-success -rate-of-aa.

2. Corrie MacLaggan, "In Texas, Less Progress on Curbing Teen Pregnancy," *Texas Tribune*, July 6, 2014, https://www.texastribune.org/2014/07/06/ teen-births-texas/.

3. Power to Decide, "Teen Birth Rate Comparison, 2020," accessed February 19, 2023, https://powertodecide.org/what-we-do/information/national -state-data/teen-birth-rate.

Chapter 29: It's Happening

1. Megan Brenan, "Record High in U.S. Put Off Medical Care Due to Cost in 2022," Gallup, January 17, 2023, https://news.gallup.com/poll/468053/ record-high-put-off-medical-care-due-cost-2022.aspx.

2. National Multiple Sclerosis Society, "Socioeconomic Factors Linked to Vision and Mental Health in People with MS, Says New Research Funded by Society," December 29, 2021, https://www .nationalmssociety.org/About-the-Society/News/Socioeconomic -Factors-Linked-to-Vision-and-Mental.

Chapter 33: A Near Miss

1. Martin Makary and Michael Daniel, "Medical Error—the Third Leading Cause of Death in the US," *BMJ* 353 (May 3, 2016): i2139, doi:10.1136/ bmj.i2139.

Epilogue

1. Munira Z. Gunja, Evan D. Gumas, and Reginald D. Williams II, "U.S. Health Care from a Global Perspective, 2022: Accelerating Spending, Worsening Outcomes," Commonwealth Fund, January 31, 2023, https:// doi.org/10.26099/8ejy-yc74.

Acknowledgments

To those who helped bring this book to life, I am forever indebted: my thoughtful, persistent, and encouraging agent, Lisa Hagan; my exceptionally talented and patient editor, Darcie Abbene, and the entire team at Health Communications, Inc.; my writing coach and book whisperer, the incomparable Brenda Copeland. Others who provided wise counsel earlier in the process include Spike Gillespie; Cynthia Levinson; Becka Oliver and others at the Writers' League of Texas; Regina Ryan; and my earliest readers: Laura Grim, Hannah Levbarg, and Bob Richter. Thanks also to Lindsey Mach and Joanne McCall for guidance in reaching readers and getting this book noticed.

To the people who provided suggestions and endorsements, I so appreciate the gift of your time reviewing my manuscript, your thoughtful feedback, and kind words.

To my patients, thank you for sharing your stories and for giving me the honor of being your doctor. I have learned from you and appreciated your patience with me, as I was so often running late. I wish you good health and much happiness.

To my coworkers—Terri, Kim, Mary, Susan, Beth, Joy, Ruperta, Hilda, Jo Linda, Naomi, Shannon, Majid, Charles, Terin, Natali, Daniela, Monica, Laura, and all the others who joined our team over the years—I enjoyed our time working together and treasure our shared memories. I hope that I've done justice to the story of our special little clinic, though I regret that I couldn't include each of you in it.

To my MS neurologist, my other doctors, and their caring staff, thanks for your compassion and brilliance. I can still work, travel, run, raise my kids, and so much more, in large part, because of you.

To my MS community—Lisa Sailor; Lisa Steffek and all of Team Tacodeli; other Texas MS150 riders; Dr. Leorah Freeman; Amie Jean; Sheldon Metz; the National MS Society, especially the South Central Board; and so many others—I am strengthened and inspired by your commitment to improving the lives of people living with MS. Getting to know many of you has been a shiny silver lining to my MS diagnosis. Together, we will eventually end MS forever!

To the people across Texas and the United States who are striving to improve healthcare access and quality, to reduce barriers and reach those who have been left out, don't give up. Your work is vital. You are saving lives and getting us closer to an inclusive, compassionate system like we all deserve.

To my friends, who continued to at least pretend to be interested in my (slow) progress on this endless writing project, thank you for your encouragement, suggestions, and unwavering support. My life is full of fun and love thanks to each of you. A special shout-out to Jess, Laura, Hannah, Marcie, Kerry, Mary Ann, Marcia, Swati, Margaret, Anita, Sierra, Dalit, Melissa, Sally, and Rachel.

More than anything, I am thankful for my warm, generous, loving, and supportive family—the greatest blessing of my life. To Don, Ella,

Clara, my parents—Libby and Lloyd Doggett—as well as Cathy, Brian, Zayla, Canyon, Ann Marie, Don Sr., Beth, Chris, Riley, and others in my extended family who have cheered me on and supported me over the years and decades: I have written nearly one hundred thousand words in this book and still can't find language to express my appreciation. Please know that I am tremendously grateful for every one of you.

There are so many other people who have touched my life in important ways. Thank you, too, for contributing to my story.

About the Author

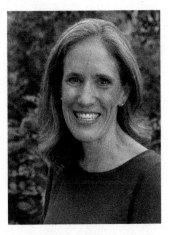

Lisa Doggett is a family physician, writer, and MS warrior based in Austin, Texas. An activist at heart, she is a cofounder of Texas Physicians for Social Responsibility and a columnist for *Public Health Watch*. She previously directed a safety-net clinic where she saw a mix of patients struggling with their own health challenges in a deeply dysfunctional system. She has battled frustrating symptoms, relapses, and insurance companies. But she has also run two marathons and completed a Half Ironman triathlon, traveled throughout the U.S. and internationally, raised two daughters, and embraced her work as a physician leader dedicated to improving health care for underserved communities.

Lisa graduated from Amherst College, Baylor College of Medicine, and the University of Texas School of Public Health. She has been published in the *New York Times*, the *Dallas Morning News*, *Motherwell*, the *Seattle Post-Intelligencer*, the *Austin American-Statesman*, and on NPR.org. She blogs for the National MS Society's *Momentum* magazine and has been featured in *Parents* magazine, *Women's World*, and on *CBS Sunday Morning*. She lives near downtown Austin, with her husband, Don Williams, a hospital-based pediatrician, and their two daughters, Ella and Clara. This is her first book. For more, please visit her website: www.lisadoggett.com.